CONQUER BACK AND NECK PAIN:

Walk It Off!

MARK D. BROWN, MD, PhD

hairman Emeritus, Department of Orthopaedics and Rehabilitation, University of Miami Miller School of Medicine

Foreword by Dr. James Weinstein,

Editor-in-Chief, SPINE, the most frequently cited and read spine journal in the world.

SUNRISE River Press

All reasonable effort has been made to assure the accuracy of the information in this book. However, this information is not meant to be all inclusive or to be a substitute for direct diagnosis and treatment by a qualified physician. Readers who have questions about a particular condition or possible treatments for that condition are advised to consult with a physician. The author and the publisher shall not be liable for any damages allegedly arising from the information in this book. The opinions expressed in this book are the author's alone and not those of the publisher. Whenever a person can be identified in this book, either they or a surviving family member gave permission to the author for their story to be told in an effort to help you.

Library of Congress Cataloging-in-Publication Data

Brown, Mark D.

Conquer back and neck pain : walk it off! a spine doctor's proven solutions for finding relief without pills or surgery / Mark D. Brown.

p. cm.

ISBN 978-1-934716-01-4

1. Backache--Popular works. 2. Neck pain--Popular works. I. Title.

RD771.B217.B758 2008

617.5'6--dc22

2007049940

ISBN 978-1-934716-47-2

SRP601P

SUNRISE River Press

39966 Grand Avenue

North Branch, MN 55056 USA

(651) 277-1400 or (800) 895-4585

TABLE OF CONTENTS

TABLE OF CONTENTS

FOREWORD

In *Conquer Back and Neck Pain: Walk It Off!* Dr. Mark Brown brings more than 35 years of clinical and research experience to those of us who are interested in the challenges presented by these most common of musculoskeletal maladies. Dr. Brown has been an international leader in this most important area of healthcare, and we can all benefit from his compassionate approach to his patients.

Back and neck pain are without a doubt the nemesis of the musculoskeletal aliments and account for nearly 100 million episodes per year just in the U.S., with 62 million having back symptoms and 21 million reporting neck symptoms. The impact is realized not only in number of visits to a multitude of healthcare providers, but also in lost productivity as a nation. Back pain accounts for the greatest number of days lost from work, making up the largest part of some $800 million (direct medical and indirect, work- and home-related) spent annually on musculoskeletal conditions. Lost workdays are most commonly due to low back pain, averaging almost one day per month per injured worker.

As a true clinician scientist, Dr. Brown provides real-life experiences to enlighten us all. He is the consummate patient advocate who presents us with a practical, no-nonsense approach to the diagnosis and treatment of back and neck pain.

Dr. Brown's seven types of neck and back pain remind me of Stephen Covey's seven habits of highly effective people. Covey allows each of us to take more control of our hectic lives and allows us to spend more time in quadrants that are effective and meaningful. Dr. Brown allows us to classify our symptoms in a way that makes understanding our condition and what to do about it simple and yet doesn't underestimate the symptoms' impact on our lives or those of our families, who need to understand what is wrong, what isn't wrong, and what to do to get better. He helps us to understand how we can take responsibility in a partnership with our doctor and to know "when to walk it off" and "when to call for help."

The role of your family doctor has never been more important, and in most cases he or she is the best front-line diagnostician and your advocate. As an advocate for shared decision-making, or what we at the Dartmouth Institute call "informed choice," Dr. Brown empowers patients with evidence-based knowledge while understanding their values and preferences, serving as a true exemplar of a patient advocate. Dr. Brown's book should be on the bookshelves in each primary care physician's office and serve as a partner to those on the front lines.

What's your activity level? Are you a couch potato, a weekend warrior, an avid runner, or – like me – somewhere in between? Dr. Brown's activity groupings allow us to understand where we are and what we can expect or need to do to change our expectations. Finally, Dr. Brown allows us to be who we are but to challenge ourselves to be better for ourselves, our partners, our families, our friends, and colleagues in the workplace. He teaches us how to be the ruler of our own back and neck symptoms and how not to be ruled by them. He advocates for surgery in special circumstances, and those need to be clear and better understood by all of us. By reading this book we can benefit from Dr. Brown's years of experience and thousands of patient visits summarized so succinctly in this book.

The patient testimonials say it all. Thank you, Dr. Brown, I can *Conquer Back and Neck Pain: Walk It Off!*

Dr. James N. Weinstein

Director, The Dartmouth Institute for Health Policy and Clinical Practice
Chairman, The Department of Orthopaedics,
Dartmouth Medical School, Dartmouth Hitchock Medical Center
Editor-in-Chief, *SPINE* (the most frequently cited and read spine journal in the world)

ABOUT THE AUTHOR

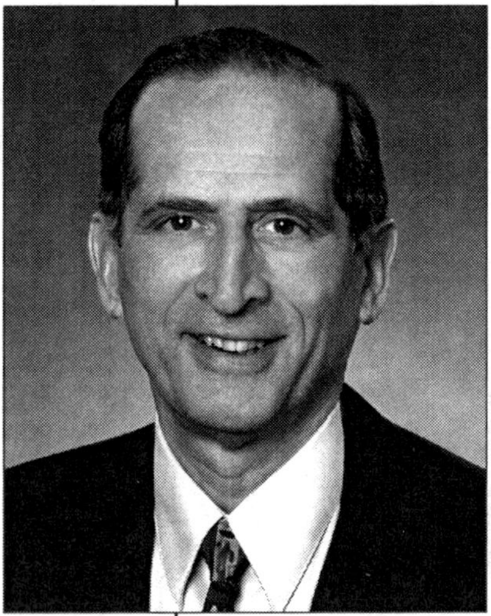

Mark D. Brown is Professor and Chairman Emeritus of the Department of Orthopaedics and Rehabilitation, University of Miami Miller School of Medicine. He has been a practicing spine surgeon for 35+ years, with his Ph.D. thesis and all of his research being devoted to the cause, prevention, and cure of painful spinal disorders. He is a founding member of the International Society for the Study of Lumbar Spine, and his other memberships include the American Academy of Orthopaedic Surgery, American Orthopaedic Association, Association of Bone and Joint Surgeons, the Cervical Spine Research Society, and the North American Spine Society. He serves as a Consultant Reviewer for the Journal of Bone and Joint Surgery, on the Board of Associate Editors of Clinical Orthopaedics and Related Research, the Associate Editorial Board of Spine, and the Editorial Board of Journal of Spinal Disorders & Techniques.

ACKNOWLEDGMENTS

It is because of my patients that I have written this book. I thank them for the honor of treating them and inspiring me to write about their problems in order to help you.

I thank all of the patients and families who have allowed me to share their stories in this book, also in order to help you.

From its inception, Tom Sand, of Health Communications, Inc., has believed in the important message of this book. He gave me valuable advice from the perspective of

This book is dedicated to my fellow back pain sufferers…may they find lasting relief.

a patient as well as a seasoned publisher. He introduced me to a number of people in the book business, one of whom is Roanne Weismann, a health care writer, who introduced me to Sunrise River Press, and Karin Hill, my editor. Karin's work ethic and editing skills are apparent in the quality of this book. Although we have never met in person, but know each other over the phone and on-line, she has become a friend for life. It has been a lot of fun editing this book with her.

Those members of my family who are more sophisticated in writing than I am helped me get my message across. I am particularly grateful to my wife, Josie, my brother, Thom, and Chris and Tony, my sons, for agonizing over many iterations of the manuscript. Rebecca, my niece and a book author, introduced me to Mike Marland, the great cartoonist who illustrated this book.

Special thanks are due to teachers and professional colleagues, two of whom, during their lives, were particularly influential to my understanding of the problem of back pain. My professor of orthopaedics, Dr. Anthony De Palma, encouraged me to become an orthopedic surgeon as well as to write a Ph.D. thesis on disc degeneration. He instilled in me a desire to study the problem of back pain throughout my career. Dr. Alf Nachemson, a fellow founding member of the International Society for the Study of the Lumbar Spine, taught me to only prescribe treatments for back pain that have been proven in well-designed clinical research trials.

I have named only a few of the people who have influenced me to present this important information to you. Although many others who helped me on this book remain anonymous, their contributions were important, and I am grateful to them. They know who they are.

INTRODUCTION

Since you're reading this, you're probably getting tired of struggling with back pain. You may have tried many types of treatments already, but so far nothing has helped. You may be starting to wonder if surgery is the only option that will finally let you reclaim a pain-free life.

If you search the Internet for information on "back pain," you will quickly find out that you are not the only one whose back hurts. In fact, back pain is so common that it seems everyone has had it at one time or another. But there are many different types of back pain, and hundreds of ways to treat it, so how are you to know what's causing your back pain, and what you should do about it?

In my more than 35 years of studying back pain and treating patients suffering with it, I have developed an approach to treatment and prevention that I recommend to everyone I treat. My approach is safe, effective, as painless as it can be, and less expensive than most other approaches!

It has been proven in medical studies that an understanding of the problem is half the cure.

Not a day goes by without a patient saying, "Thank you, doctor, for explaining what I have, what to expect, and what my options are for relief. I feel better already!" This book contains the same advice I give my patients: down-to-earth explanations of what is wrong, what to expect, how to get relief, and how to prevent the pain from recurring. It has been proven in medical studies that an understanding of the problem is half the cure. The object of this book is to give you: 1) an understanding of the seven types of back pain; 2) a way to determine which type is affecting you; and 3) information on what really works to prevent and cure your pain.

There are many astonishing "treatments" described on the Internet that I don't recommend, either because they are not proven to work, they do not provide lasting relief, or because they are dangerous compared to safer and less expensive alternatives. And, although surgery is certainly necessary in some cases of back pain, I have found that the vast majority of problems are cured without surgery. People often get frustrated after trying numerous treatments and painkillers that don't solve their problem, and they conclude that surgery is their only option for relief. What they don't realize is that it's often the very treatments they think should be helping them that actually *hinder* their own body's efforts to heal! In this book, I will tell you what treatments to avoid and why they may be making you worse.

I'll also give you stories of real-life back-pain sufferers. These people have agreed to tell you their stories in the hope that their experiences will help you. You may very well recognize your own problem in one of these stories and realize that you are not alone. You will read how other people with a problem similar to yours found out what was wrong, how they found relief, and how they avoid recurrent attacks of pain.

There are many myths surrounding back pain, such as: we have it because we walk upright; it is all in your mind; specific back exercises will relieve it; and good posture will prevent it from happening. However, the facts are a bit different: most back pain is genetic; it's really your back and not your mind; back-specific exercises may aggravate it; and good posture does not entirely prevent you from having an attack of back pain. I will explain why these myths, and others, are not helpful in understanding why you suffer from back pain, and how believing in some of them may be keeping you from getting better.

Rarely should back pain keep you from doing the things you enjoy, like golf and sex. We do not have to suffer from it as much as we do. I will explain when to worry and when not to worry about your pain, when to "walk if off," when to run (hobble) for medical help, and what treatments to avoid that may actually make your pain worse!

CHAPTER 1

Back Pain Is Very Common, and Here's Why

Every year I am asked to give a lecture on back pain to the senior class of the University of Miami's nationally recognized Physical Therapy School. I start out the lecture by asking the students, the majority of whom are under the age of 30, "Raise your hand if you have suffered from back pain severe enough to have warranted seeing a doctor?" Much to my amazement, each time I ask these young people, more than 50 percent of them raise their hand. This is true year in and year out. Back pain is an epidemic in modern societies, affecting more than 80 percent of people at one time or another during their life. Back pain is allegedly second only to the common cold as a reason for time lost from work. Everyone knows someone who has suffered from back pain. But what causes back pain? Why is it so common? Before answering these questions, let's look at one other interesting aspect of back pain. Even though it is so common, it is rarely serious.

Back pain is allegedly second only to the common cold as a reason for time lost from work.

My father suffered intermittent severe bouts of back pain that would render him helpless — an unusual state for him — for a day or two at a time. I recall that he would take aspirin, rest for a few hours to allow the acute spasms to subside, then — slowly, gingerly, painfully, and crookedly — get out of bed and walk it off!

As he got older his attacks occurred less frequently and were less severe. It wasn't until years later that I would understand why he had these attacks and why they became less frequent as he aged. I would also learn how he could have prevented the frequency and severity of the attacks that he suffered from, through exercise and a healthier lifestyle.

His sister, my aunt, was not as lucky as he was. She suffered from neck pain for many years, and while I was in medical school she began to develop terrible symptoms of loss of balance and aching throughout her body. She went from doctor to doctor, but none could determine what was wrong, and a few of them labeled her neurotic.

One day while I was visiting her she described her symptoms and frustration with the medical advice she had received. I coincidentally had just rotated on the world-famous neurology service at Thomas Jefferson Medical School, where I had learned how to diagnose myelopathy, a disease of the spinal cord that causes loss of balance, stumbling, aches and pains in the arms and legs, and propensity to fall. I recognized her symptoms and arranged for her to see my neurology professor. He performed a myelogram, a test in which x-ray contrast dye is injected into the spinal canal, and confirmed that my aunt had pressure on her spinal cord from spinal stenosis (constriction of the spinal canal). She underwent surgery to relieve the pressure on her spinal cord, but her condition was too advanced and she subsequently died from complications of progressive paralysis. I was devastated by how this could have happened to her and vowed to determine how it did and what could have been done to prevent it!

As I was to discover later, my father's back pain and my aunt's spinal cord disease had been related to the same phenomenon: disc degeneration. Disc degeneration is a condition in which the normal cushioning function of the spinal disc is lost through the aging process, and it leads to spinal pain in a variety of ways. What I learned about disc degeneration, the most common cause of back pain, will help you understand what may be happening to you to cause your neck, back, arm, or leg pain.

To be human is to have neck and back pain

One of the things that I have learned is that it is not our fault that we have back pain; it is because we are human! The first myth concerning back pain is that we have it because we walk upright on two feet. Wrong! Man's best friend, our loveable pooch, who walks on all four legs, is as likely to have back pain as we are. On the other hand, our feline friends, cats, are not! It seems that back pain, slipped discs, spinal stenosis, and arthritis of the spine are the bane of people and dogs, but not cats. And the reason for this is in our genetic code and how it programs our discs to age before the rest of our body. We are just beginning to learn that conditions that cause back pain are more common in some species than in others. Unfortunately, we are one of those species that are susceptible to back pain.

One of my professors told me of a humorous conversation he had with one of his patients. The patient complained about the surgical fee my professor charged him to perform a disc excision. He wasn't upset that the fee was too high; rather, he thought it was too low! It seems that the patient had paid a higher fee to a veterinarian to perform a disc excision on his dachshund than the professor had charged the gentleman

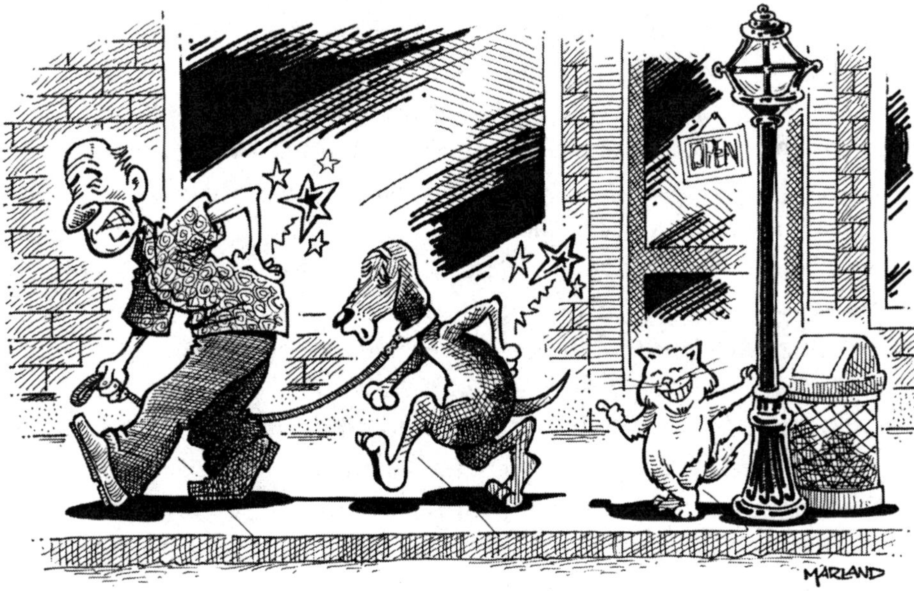

for his own disc surgery. I tell you this story only to illustrate that we share our susceptibility to disc herniation with our canine pals. Misery loves company!

The bad news is that most of us do have the genetic makeup for disc degeneration, which leads to painful back disorders. The good news is that, unlike our canine pals, we can do something to keep these disorders from hurting and harming us.

Back pain is not our fault; we are programmed to get it because we belong to the human species. But, unlike other species, we can do something about it! First let us look at why we are genetically predisposed to painful spinal conditions so that we can understand how to prevent back pain and how it will be treated in the future.

Genetics, back pain, and disc degeneration

The discs in our spine are genetically programmed to prematurely age, degenerate, or deteriorate, however you want to describe the phenomenon. This can occur as early as in our 20s! It is not unusual for me to see a teenager suffering from back pain that is caused by a prematurely aged disc. I wondered why this should be, so I asked one of my students to analyze the family histories of an unusual group of 63 young people who, by the age of 21, had undergone surgery for a herniated "slipped" disc. We then compared them to the family histories of another group of 63 people of the same age and sex who never had a history of back pain or disc problems. A significant number of relatives of the symptomatic youth had a history of back pain or herniated disc compared to the families of the group of young people who never had symptoms. Genetic experts interpreted these findings as strong evidence for an inherited susceptibility to back pain and disc herniation. We published these findings in the medical literature.

Subsequent clinical studies of adults have provided further evidence of a genetic basis for spinal disc degeneration in humans, as well as the relationship between disc-degeneration back pain and disc herniation. In the final chapter of this book we will explore the current research into how to replace the defective genes that cause discs to age before the rest of our body in order to prevent back pain.

Why does our genetic makeup cause the discs in our body to age before the rest of us? How does aging of the disc cause pain? In order to answer these questions, we must first look at how a normal disc is made and how it functions.

How do spinal discs work?

The 23 discs in our body are positioned between the vertebrae (the bone blocks that support your spine) and are firmly attached to them. They cushion our spine and yet allow our spine to move in all directions. The center of each disc is composed of a gelatinous tissue that functions like a sponge (nucleus pulposus) that soaks up water so strongly that it is hard to squeeze it out. The firmly held water in the center of the disc distributes the weight of your body evenly against your vertebrae much the same way that air in an automobile tire distributes the weight of your car on the road.

Your spinal discs are living structures that contain cells that produce and maintain the nucleus pulposus. Since there are no blood vessels in the disc, the cells depend on diffusion to move nutrients into the disc and waste out of the disc through the nucleus pulposus, which the cells themselves produce and maintain. If something impairs the flow of nutrients into the disc, the cells will get sick and begin to die off. The nucleus will break down and no longer hold water as tightly in the disc, and the disc will deflate. The concept of the disc as a living structure with cells that produce a gel-like center that holds water will be important to understand in Chapter 11, where we explore how to keep your discs in good shape and prevent back pain from occurring.

As you walk around during the day, the weight of your body normally squeezes some of the water out of your discs and you get shorter. During a good night's sleep, normal discs suck up the water again and you become taller by morning. This is important for the health of your disc, but it's a big problem for astronauts. In the weightless environment of space, spinal discs swell so much that they can actually fracture the attached vertebrae and cause back pain. Back on earth the same thing can happen to you if you are forced to spend too much time in bed. More will be said about this in Chapter 11.

What makes the discs break down?

So what does all of this mean with respect to back pain? A number of genes have been identified that control the way the cells make and maintain the sponge in our discs. When we are missing a few of these genes, the cells are programmed to make a sponge that does not hold the water tightly enough to allow the disc to function properly. Not only does the disc cushion poorly, but food cannot get into the cells in the disc and waste cannot get out. The cells get sick and eventually die and the disc begins to literally fall apart, or degenerate. When this happens the disc cannot bear weight properly and begins to narrow.

How does a disc that is falling apart cause pain?

Picture the situation where you are driving down the street and you notice that one of the tires on the car in front of you is half flat. You are most likely compelled to drive up alongside of the car, blow your horn to get the driver's attention, lower the window of your car, and warn the driver of the condition of their tire. Why? Because you know that there is not enough air in the tire to distribute the weight of the car properly and you are afraid that a half-flat tire may blow out and cause an accident.

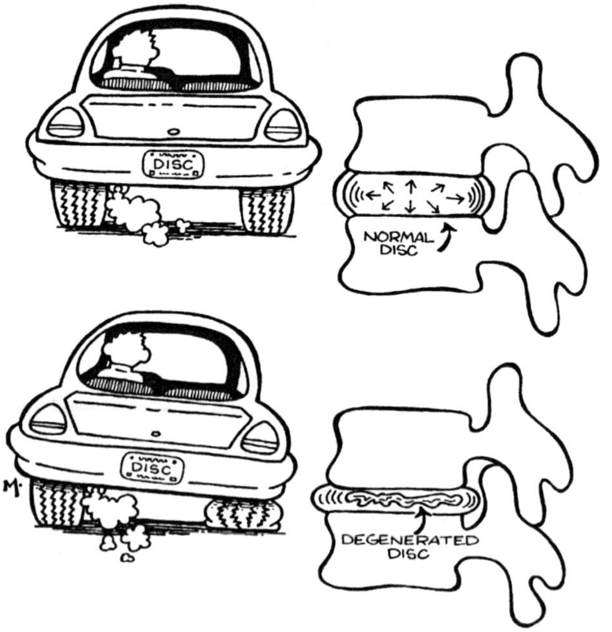

The same thing happens when a disc degenerates. The loss of water in the center of the degenerated disc causes it to deflate and lose its ability to cushion. Abnormal weight is placed on the tough side wall of the disc (annulus fibrosus) and it breaks down. Initially, tears in the side wall of the disc are not felt because there are no nerves in the disc itself. But when the tears reach the nerve endings in the surrounding tissues, back pain may occur. When tears go completely through the rim of the disc, the spongy center of the disc may herniate completely through the tear in the side wall and compress the adjacent nerve to produce leg or arm pain.

Sometimes the center spongy part of the disc becomes so degenerated and dried out that it cannot squeeze through the tears in the rim of the disc to cause back and extremity pain. This is an important concept to understand, so I'll explain in the next few paragraphs how disc degeneration is detected and how we know it sometimes causes pain and at other times does not.

Disc degeneration: the ultimate culprit for back pain

Since the development of MRI scans (see how MRI works on page 52) we can clearly see the extent of spinal disc degeneration without the need for any injections or x-ray exposure. MRI scans have been used in population studies and have shown that there is some degree of disc degeneration present in almost every adult, whether they have a history of back pain or not.

Some medical scientists say that disc degeneration is not the cause of back pain. They draw this conclusion because several classic MRI studies have revealed disc degeneration in people who had never experienced back pain. Yes, there really are a fortunate few! The incidence of disc degeneration detected on the MRI scans of these fortunate individuals is not much different from that in a group of people who have suffered from back pain. So, some medical experts have used these studies to debunk the disc as the source of back pain. I and other spinal experts disagree with them; we interpret the results of these studies to mean that disc degeneration may or may not result in pain, and that people with disc degeneration but no back pain at the time of the MRI scan are likely to develop pain related to it in the future.

In other studies using discography (injection of x-ray dye into the disc to determine the degree of degeneration and to stimulate back pain), it has been shown that some discs become pain stimulators during the course of degenerating and some do not. Performing discography on the same disc at different times has also shown that some discs may be painful at one stage of degeneration but not in a later stage of degeneration. This concept is important in understanding how it is possible to obtain relief from chronic back pain (Chapter 8).

There are four ways that disc degeneration can cause back and/or extremity pain:

- through pressure on a spinal nerve from a disc herniation or from constriction of the spinal canal (neurogenic pain)
- through susceptibility to sprains and strains (mechanical pain)
- through leakage of painful breakdown products of the disc itself (discogenic pain)
- when disc degeneration results in deformity of the spine such as curvature (scoliosis), it may result in muscle-fatigue pain

When disc material actually herniates into the spinal canal it can compress and irritate the spinal nerves, which can result in pain in the extremities. Shakespeare, in the play *Timon of Athens*, 1564, described "thou cold sciatica crippled our senators that their limbs may halt as lamely as their manners." Sciatica is a pain that travels down the back of the legs along the course of the sciatic nerve and is usually caused by a disc herniation in the low back (lumbar spine). Disc herniations in the neck (cervical spine) can cause pain in the arms; disc herniations in the spine behind the chest (thoracic spine) can cause pain in the chest and abdomen.

The late stages of disc degeneration result in deflation of the disc and bulging of the outer rim. When this occurs, narrowing of the spinal canal and nerve channels may result. This is called spinal stenosis. If the narrowing of the spinal canal results in compression of the spinal nerves, back and extremity pain may result. My aunt's demise was caused by spinal stenosis in her neck, which in addition to pain resulted in compression of her spinal cord and paralysis. I will devote an entire chapter to the subject of spinal stenosis since it is the most common cause of neck, back, and extremity pain as we get older – yet most people have never even heard of it!

As discs become progressively degenerated, they may become unstable and susceptible to repeated painful sprains from the stress of normal activity. This is a common cause of chronic mechanical lower-back pain. I will discuss the consequences of the late stages of disc degeneration, how to prevent them, and how to get relief from them in several chapters of this book.

In the final stages of disc degeneration the discs begin to stiffen up to the point that they become functionally fused together by bone spurs, called osteophytes, on the margins of the vertebrae. This is a normal healing process by the body in response to repeated small sprains of the disc when it is not bearing weight properly during the early stages of disc degeneration. The bone spurs that form at the attachment of the disc to the vertebral bodies act to stabilize the disc. However, bone spurs from disc degeneration may contribute to narrowing of the spinal nerve channels and cause nerve pain. More will be said about this in Chapter 6 on spinal stenosis.

Disc degeneration may result in slippage of the spine (spondylolisthesis), curvature of the spine (scoliosis), and/or a bent spine (kyphosis). Any one or a combination of these deformities can throw the spine off balance. The normal reflexes in your body will try to keep your head centered over your pelvis. When the spine is out of balance, these reflexes make the muscles continuously work to correct the deformity. As a result, the muscles fatigue and become painful.

During the course of disc degeneration, the breakdown products of the tissues may themselves become irritants and leak through cracks in the sidewall of the disc to cause inflammation in the surrounding nerve endings. The pain that results can come and go without warning or apparent cause. Pain resulting from irritating breakdown products of a degenerated disc is difficult to diagnose and to treat. It will be discussed throughout this book, especially in the chapter on chronic back pain.

Through an understanding that disc degeneration is genetic, ubiquitous in humans, and responsible for the majority of painful conditions of the spine and extremities, I developed a strategy for diagnosis, treatment, and prevention of spine pain. The strategy will be presented in the following chapters. Referring back to this chapter as needed, I will give you a better understanding of how to obtain relief from back pain and how to keep your back pain from recurring.

The next chapter will describe the seven types of neck and back pain and includes a questionnaire to help you determine the type(s) of pain that you have. You can use this questionnaire as a guide to various types of spine pain in the remaining chapters.

CHAPTER 2

Which of the 7 Types of Back Pain Do You Have?

The seven types of neck and back pain are:

1. **Nerve root pain** from compression and irritation of a spinal nerve by a herniated spinal disc
2. **Neurogenic pain** caused by loss of oxygen to the spinal nerves by constriction of the spinal canal (spinal stenosis) and/or smoking
3. **Mechanical pain**, caused by an unstable spine from an injury or defect such as spondylolisthesis (slippage of the spine)
4. **Chemical or discogenic pain** from breakdown products of a degenerated disc
5. **Muscle fatigue pain** from an out-of-balance deformity such as curvature or slippage of the spine
6. **Inflammatory pain** such as from arthritis or infection of the spine
7. **Central pain** resulting from a low threshold to pain, secondary to depression and/or narcotic-induced depletion of endorphins

It is important to know what type of neck and back pain you are suffering from, because the treatment and prevention of recurrence will differ depending on the type.

Neck and back pain conditions are usually the result of some combination of these types acting at the same time. In the first phases of disc degeneration, mechanical pain from a loose disc may predominate. In later stages of disc degeneration, the primary discomfort may be chemical pain from irritating breakdown products of the disc. A herniated disc may cause nerve root pain by stretching and compressing an adjacent spinal nerve, whereas a collapsed bulging disc may cause constriction of the spinal nerve channels (spinal stenosis), resulting in neurogenic pain. Inflammatory pain may come from a disc-space infection or from one of several forms of inflammatory arthritis that affect the disc, such as rheumatoid arthritis and ankylosing spondylitis. Pain that is experienced as the result of faulty central (brain) pain modulating systems is usually secondary to depression and/or depletion of our body's own natural pain killers – our endorphins – by narcotics or muscle relaxants.

It is important to know what type of neck and back pain you are suffering from, because the treatment and prevention of recurrence will differ depending on the type. Treatment for one type of pain may make another type of pain worse: painkillers for nerve pain may make central pain worse, and disc excision to treat neurogenic pain may cause the disc to collapse further and exacerbate spinal stenosis and neurogenic pain.

How do you know what type of neck and/or back pain is causing you to suffer? The following questionnaire is made up of statements or questions that are grouped into the seven types of pain. If you answer most of the questions yes in one group you are probably suffering from that type of pain. However, it is also possible that you are suffering from more than one type of pain at the same time. Let us begin the quiz.

1) Nerve root pain

If you answer most of these questions with a yes, then you most likely are suffering from nerve root pain from a herniated disc:

- I have pain from my low back down the back of my leg, down the front of my leg, or from my neck into my arm. ❑Yes ❑No
- The pain in my leg or arm is associated with numbness, tingling, pins and needles, or other bothersome sensations. ❑Yes ❑No

- I have difficulty sleeping because of the pain. ❑Yes ❑No
- The pain in my leg causes me to limp. ❑Yes ❑No
- The pain makes my knee give out or makes my ankle weak. ❑Yes ❑No
- The pain in my arm causes me to lose my grip on things. ❑Yes ❑No
- The pain in my leg is worse when I lean forward while I am standing. ❑Yes ❑No
- I can clearly describe where the pain is in my leg or my arm. ❑Yes ❑No
- Raising my arm on my head somewhat relieves my arm pain. ❑Yes ❑No
- Lying on my back with my hip and knee bent relieves my leg pain. ❑Yes ❑No

If you answered most of these questions with a yes, then you might want to go to Chapter 5 to learn more about herniated discs and other conditions that can cause these symptoms.

2) Neurogenic pain

You may be suffering from neurogenic pain from constriction of the spinal canal (spinal stenosis) if you answer the majority of these statements/questions with a yes:

- Aching pain in my legs keeps me from walking as far as I want to walk. ❑Yes ❑No
- The aching in my legs goes away as soon as I sit, and then I can walk again. ❑Yes ❑No
- I can swim, dance, or bicycle, but I cannot walk because of pain. ❑Yes ❑No
- I tend to walk better when I lean on something like a shopping cart. ❑Yes ❑No
- When I bend forward I can walk further without leg pain. ❑Yes ❑No
- My arm aches when I am writing, but the pain goes away when I stop. ❑Yes ❑No

- I can walk further some days than others. ❑Yes ❑No
- I can bend over and my legs feel better. ❑Yes ❑No
- I tend to stumble, trip, or fall more than before. ❑Yes ❑No
- My walking is unsteady. ❑Yes ❑No

If these are your symptoms, you can read more about spinal stenosis and neurogenic pain in Chapter 6.

3) Mechanical pain

A yes to most of these questions means you are suffering from mechanical neck or back pain:

- Lifting anything heavier than a quart (liter) of milk bothers my back. ❑Yes ❑No
- Twisting and bending can bring on an attack of back pain. ❑Yes ❑No
- I have back pain when I first change position, such as when standing up after sitting. ❑Yes ❑No
- My back can go out from the smallest thing. ❑Yes ❑No
- Leaning back bothers my back. ❑Yes ❑No
- A corset, brace, or neck collar gives me relief. ❑Yes ❑No
- Turning my head or looking up bothers my neck. ❑Yes ❑No
- Lying down relieves my back or neck pain for a while. ❑Yes ❑No

More about mechanical back pain can be found in Chapter 7 on injuries and deformity of the spine, and in Chapter 8 on chronic back pain.

4) Chemical or discogenic pain

Answering yes to most of the following questions could mean you are experiencing chemical or discogenic pain – pain arising from a disc that is leaking irritating breakdown products. This type of pain is difficult to distinguish from nerve root and mechanical pain and frequently occurs along with these types of pain:

- My neck or back pain comes and goes without reason. ❑Yes ❑No
- Anti-inflammatory medications give me some relief. ❑Yes ❑No
- The less active I am, the more it seems to hurt. ❑Yes ❑No

- The pain sometimes keeps me from falling asleep, but once I am asleep I am OK. ❑Yes ❑No
- Pain medicines don't seem to make any difference. ❑Yes ❑No

Learn more about chemical discogenic pain in Chapter 8 on chronic back pain.

5) Muscle fatigue pain

Characteristics of muscle fatigue pain from spinal deformity, which causes your spine to be out of balance, can be discerned from these statements/questions:

- I have difficulty standing straight. ❑Yes ❑No
- I feel as if my spine is out of balance. ❑Yes ❑No
- I feel like I am leaning like the Tower of Pisa. ❑Yes ❑No
- I feel like one hip is higher than the other. ❑Yes ❑No
- People say I look crooked. ❑Yes ❑No
- I feel as if I am tilted forward. ❑Yes ❑No

For more about this type of pain go to Chapter 7 on spinal deformity.

6) Inflammatory pain

Inflammation from arthritis can cause symptoms that are acute or chronic. Here are some statements/questions you can answer to determine if you have this type of pain:

- My back feels stiff when I get up in the morning. ❑Yes ❑No
- It takes me several hours to limber up in the morning. ❑Yes ❑No
- Anti-inflammatory medication helps me function better with the pain. ❑Yes ❑No
- I have rheumatoid arthritis and my neck hurts. ❑Yes ❑No
- I have arthritis in my other joints. ❑Yes ❑No
- I have a history of osteoarthritis. ❑Yes ❑No
- My spine flexibility is getting worse as I get older. ❑Yes ❑No

Learn more about inflammation, arthritis, and infection of the spine in both the chapters on acute and chronic back pain, Chapters 3 and 8.

7) Central pain

You may be suffering from some component of central pain if you answer yes to most of the following statements:

- The pain medicine I take does not seem to work any more. ❑Yes ❑No
- It takes more and stronger pain medication for me to get relief. ❑Yes ❑No
- I have been on narcotic pain medication and/or muscle relaxants for more than one month. ❑Yes ❑No
- I must take a sleeping pill to sleep. ❑Yes ❑No
- I feel depressed because of my pain. ❑Yes ❑No
- I suffered from depression before this pain began. ❑Yes ❑No
- The pain makes me cry a lot. ❑Yes ❑No
- My pain is controlling my life. ❑Yes ❑No
- I have pain all over my body. ❑Yes ❑No

For more about central pain and chronic back pain see Chapter 8.

Other, serious causes of pain requiring immediate medical attention

The following groups of statements are to help you determine if your spine pain is related to some serious underlying disorder.

Cauda equina syndrome *(see page 30)*

If you answer yes to the majority of the following questions, you may be suffering from pressure on the nerves to your legs, bladder, and bowel. This is a serious condition called cauda equina syndrome, and you should seek medical attention immediately:

- I have severe back pain radiating into both legs. ❑Yes ❑No
- I am having difficulty walking because of severe back and leg pain. ❑Yes ❑No
- I am losing my urine, dribbling, and I do not feel it. ❑Yes ❑No

- I have difficulty passing my urine. ❑Yes ❑No
- I do not think I am emptying my bladder completely when I urinate. ❑Yes ❑No
- I feel numb around my genitals and anus. ❑Yes ❑No
- My legs feel weak and/or numb. ❑Yes ❑No
- This back pain makes me constipated and I am not taking pain medication. ❑Yes ❑No

To read more about this syndrome, turn to page 30.

Spine tumor

The following statements concern the symptoms of a tumor in your spine. If these statements pertain to you then you may have a tumor in your spine and you should seek medical care as soon as possible:

- Back pain awakens me every night and it is getting worse. ❑Yes ❑No
- Once the pain awakens me I must get up and walk around before I can get back to sleep. ❑Yes ❑No
- My legs seem to give out when I have the pain. ❑Yes ❑No
- I cannot sleep at all because of the pain. ❑Yes ❑No
- Any time I lie down the pain gets worse. ❑Yes ❑No

Spine infection

If you answer most of the following questions with a yes, then you may have an infection causing your spine pain:

- I have spine pain after I had an infection (urinary tract, dental, skin abscess). ❑Yes ❑No
- I am diabetic and/or on chemotherapy or on steroids. ❑Yes ❑No
- I have some other illness that suppresses my immune system. ❑Yes ❑No
- I have night sweats. ❑Yes ❑No
- I have been exposed to tuberculosis and/or have a positive tuberculin skin test. ❑Yes ❑No
- My spine pain is getting progressively worse. ❑Yes ❑No

- I have chills and fever. ❑Yes ❑No

See page 32 for more about the diagnosis and treatment of spine infections.

Constriction of the spinal canal (spinal stenosis, see Chapter 6)

The following statements may mean that you have something pressing on the spinal cord in your neck or chest. If these symptoms pertain to you, seek help as soon as possible:

- When I look up or turn my head, I become unsteady and lose my balance. ❑Yes ❑No
- If I drop my chin to my chest I get tingling sensations in my arms and/or legs. ❑Yes ❑No
- I am losing my balance lately and I must hold onto something to walk. ❑Yes ❑No
- I trip and stumble lately. ❑Yes ❑No
- I have fallen one or more times because of my balance. ❑Yes ❑No
- My hands are not as coordinated as they were in the past. ❑Yes ❑No
- My handwriting is becoming illegible. ❑Yes ❑No
- I cannot button or unbutton my shirt. ❑Yes ❑No
- I cannot climb up a curb or steps without help. ❑Yes ❑No

CHAPTER 3

Acute Severe Back Pain: What Could It Be, and What Should You Do?

Acute benign back pain

I had been working hard as Chief Resident of Orthopaedic Surgery, on call every other night, and trying to scrub in on every interesting surgical case that I could. A young man came into the emergency room with a severed nerve on the side of his knee, and he could not lift his foot up off the floor. In order to repair the nerve I had to stand in an awkward position bent forward over the operating room table for almost two hours, stitching the nerve with the aid of magnifying lenses.

The pain is horrible! What is wrong? Is it an emergency? How do I get rid of it?

In the surgeon's lounge following the operation, I bent over to put on my shoes and was struck with such a severe back pain that I almost fell to my knees. A fellow resident helped me to the emergency room, and there I was evaluated by another colleague who suspected that I was passing a kidney stone. He ordered an x-ray of my kidneys, and when the x-ray came back normal, we both realized that the pain was coming from my back. I went home and rested for a few hours with a heating pad and then got out of bed and walked it off over the next few days. I finally understood why my father was so incapacitated when he had attacks of back pain and how he recovered from what seemed to be a devastating condition by simply walking it off!

This attack was brought on by no apparent injury and went away without any real treatment except walking it off. To this day, we medical scientists have not been able to pinpoint the exact reason for such attacks of low back pain. Therefore we label the condition as idiopathic low-back pain, meaning the exact cause of the back pain is not known. I suspect such attacks of back pain represent the first complete tears in the side wall (annulus fibrosus) of a degenerated disc, tears that reach the sensitive nerve endings adjacent to the disc.

Whatever the exact reason, the vast majority of acute, severe attacks of low-back pain are way out of proportion to the seriousness of the condition that causes them, and they go away just as mysteriously – but unfortunately not as quickly – as they came. How do we know when to seek help for such an attack?

When to Walk It Off	When to Call for Help
You can still get out of bed and walk	It is too painful to walk
Your legs do not give way	Your legs are weak and won't hold you up
You have normal sensation everywhere	You have numbness in your pelvic area
You have no difficulty urinating	You cannot urinate or you lose your urine
You do not feel faint or light headed	You are faint or lightheaded
You do not feel sick	You have chills, fever, nausea, or sweating
The pain is bearable within an hour of rest	The pain is unbearable, even after rest
You do not feel anxious	The pain comes in spasms
The pain is gradually getting better	The pain is getting worse
The pain is coming from your back	You have chest or abdominal pain

When to walk it off and when to get immediate help for acute back pain

There are some simple questions you can ask yourself in order to determine whether you should seek immediate help or just walk it off like my father and I did from our attacks of back pain.

The first thing to do is lie down, relax and calm down, and try to analyze the situation. The good news is that the vast majority of acute attacks of neck and back pain are not serious enough to require emergency care. The bad news is that there are some rarely occurring serious disorders that can cause acute and severe spine pain. Therefore, if the attack of back pain is so severe that it is difficult to walk and the pain does not subside to some degree within a few hours of bed rest, then common sense dictates that you call 911 and seek emergency attention.

Benign low-back pain, also known as idiopathic low-back pain, lumbago, low-back sprain, or low-back spasm, is the most common reason for acute severe attacks of back pain. It is self-limiting, not serious, and usually will begin to subside within a few hours of onset with rest and control of the anxiety that is associated with it. You should be able to walk, although slowly, and you should be able to go to the bathroom and urinate. After the initial crescendo of pain it should begin to subside, to some degree, almost immediately.

If the pain continues to get worse, makes you faint, light headed and sweaty, and comes in spasms, you may have some other more serious condition that may endanger your life or limbs. Some conditions which may not be from your back, but that you should be aware of, are described below. Even if you have had a previous attack of severe back pain that you walked off, you should be aware of these conditions and the symptoms they produce, as they are not something to ignore if they occur.

Cauda equina syndrome, a surgical emergency

Massive disc herniation in the low back can cause cauda equina syndrome. The cauda equina (literally means horse's tail in Latin) is the term applied to the multiple nerves that go from your brain to your legs, your bowel, and your urinary bladder. If one of the lower spinal discs completely blows out, it can squash the nerves in your cauda equina, causing severe back and leg pain. If the attack of back pain is unrelenting; you experience numbness in your groin, around your rectum, genitals or legs; weakness in one or both legs; inability to urinate; or any combination of these symptoms, you should seek emergency treatment immediately! Prompt diagnosis and surgical treatment of this condition can result in a complete recovery. Fortunately, this horrible condition is responsible for less than one in 10,000 cases of severe back pain and fewer than one in 1,000 cases of disc herniation. In more than 30 years of surgical practice I have had to operate upon fewer than 10 patients with this condition, two of whom were pregnant. I will describe these two patients' cases in the chapter on disc herniation.

Acute severe back pain caused by a kidney stone

The passage of a kidney stone can cause acute severe back pain. One morning my wife complained to me of acute severe back pain while holding her side in an attempt to alleviate waves of spasmodic pain. It was obvious that she was in severe pain because she was lightheaded, sweating, and nauseous. The pain was localized to one side of her back, over her kidney just below the rib cage, and radiated into her groin area. I recognized her symptoms as those seen with passage of a kidney stone, so I took her to our emergency clinic where she was treated with medication that helped her pass the stone. Later she told me it was the most severe pain she had ever experienced, worse than giving birth. If you experience any of these symptoms, you should be seen in an emergency room. If the pain is making you lightheaded and no one is available to drive you to the emergency room, call 911. Do not try to drive yourself, as you may faint and end up in a car accident.

Vertebral fractures

Fracture of the vertebrae in the low back can cause acute severe back pain. Normal vertebrae require a significant injury to fracture (fracture and break mean the same thing), such as a fall from a ladder – one that you are sure to remember and associate with the back pain. However, there are cases in which people do not remember injuring their back, such as during a fainting attack, seizure, or while under the influence of alcohol or drugs. In instances such as these, a person may not associate severe back pain with an injury. Once again, if the pain does not subside within a few hours of resting to the point where you can get up and walk around, you need to seek help.

There are also circumstances in which one may not suspect that back pain is from a fractured spine. A defective vertebra can break from a trivial insult such as a sneeze or riding over a speed bump. Older women with soft and/or brittle bones (osteoporosis), people with unsuspected tumors in their spine, and those with chronic diseases may have defective vertebrae that are susceptible to breaking from a minor injury, thus causing severe low-back pain. For this reason, the source of any acute back pain in a frail and/or chronically ill individual should be determined by a qualified medical expert.

Shingles (herpes zoster)

Shingles is caused by the chicken pox virus. The chicken pox virus can stay dormant in your spinal nerves for years and then suddenly, within a matter of a day or two, trigger a burning, itching, acute, and chronic pain syndrome that radiates along the course of a spinal nerve anywhere in your body (head, neck, arms, trunk, legs). The pain associated with shingles may be mistaken for a herniated disc in your neck or anywhere in your back, depending on the spinal nerve affected. Shingles is characterized by a painful weepy skin rash that occurs at the site of the pain. If this occurs to you, seek immediate help from your primary care physician, a neurologist, or a dermatologist (skin specialist). There are medications available for this disease that, if given early enough, will shorten the painful course of the rash and prevent the chronic nerve pain that can develop with it.

Do not touch or scratch the rash because you can spread the virus that causes it to others or to other places on your body. It is particularly dangerous if it gets in your eye because it can injure your cornea and cause blindness! Whenever you develop burning pain associated with a skin rash, think of shingles and seek immediate help.

Painful spine infection

Bacteria from your bloodstream can spread to your spine, causing a spine infection and severe back pain. Since it is rare and may not cause fever, chills, and sweating that you would expect from an infection in other parts of your body, an infection of the spine may not initially be suspected as a cause of the pain. Diabetic patients, those undergoing chemotherapy for cancer, people who have had an organ transplant or other chronic disease, and people on steroids are more susceptible to spinal infection and should seek expert medical advice for an attack of pain involving the spine.

If you have had a recent urinary tract infection, tooth abscess, skin boil, or foot ulcer and develop severe back pain, do not forget to tell your doctor about the infection. That information will alert the doctor to the possibility that the infection has spread to your spine. Infection can spread to any disc and/or vertebra in the spine and therefore produce pain in any location of the spine: neck, thoracic, or low back. Severe pain in any of these locations in individuals who are susceptible to infection or have had a recent infection elsewhere in their body should be a warning that there could be an infection in the spine.

Aneurysm causing spine pain

An aortic aneurysm is a blowout of the major blood vessel that leads from your heart to your body. The aorta runs alongside the spine all the way from your heart to your pelvis, and a painful rupture of this blood vessel can cause back pain anywhere along your spine from your chest to your low back. This condition occurs rarely, and usually is seen in older, debilitated individuals, especially those who have a long history of smoking. But it can also be seen in young, tall, and lanky individuals, like basketball players. Some tall and thin people have a genetic condition called Marfan's Syndrome, which can be the cause of a rare form of aneurysm that can produce pain along the entire spine. Any older, deconditioned individual, man or woman, with acute back pain and/or abdominal pain should be treated on an emergency basis to rule out this life-threatening condition. The same can be said for young, tall, thin, and lanky individuals who have long, thin fingers and who complain of pain along the thoracic spine.

Acute versus recurrent and chronic back pain

When should you see a doctor for back pain that is not acute and/or severe? A good rule is to determine the cause of any back pain attack that lasts more than two weeks, as the majority of acute attacks of benign back pain get better within the first week of onset. If the attack of back pain is associated with pain radiating down an arm or leg, with numbness or weakness of the muscles, or with loss of balance, stumbling, or tripping, then you should see your doctor. Anytime an adolescent or child experiences back pain or pain in an extremity, they should be seen by a pediatrician. Children and adolescents do not complain of pain unless something is wrong. Therefore, any time they have pain they should be seen by their pediatrician. Since babies under the age of two cannot express pain verbally, you should suspect a painful condition if they scream when you touch them or try to move an arm or leg. If you suspect pain in an infant, you should take the baby to an emergency room immediately. A child of any age who has meningitis may have severe neck pain, a stiff neck, and a high temperature. Early recognition of these symptoms and prompt diagnosis and treatment can save the baby's life!

Acute neck and chest pain

Much of what I have told you about acute low-back pain is true for neck and thoracic pain, with a few important exceptions. The cervical spine (neck) is more mobile than the lumbar spine (low back) so that you can move your head normally in a range of 180 degrees from side to side and from top to bottom. The discs in your neck are subject to the same degenerative process leading to spinal pain as described above. Also, the vertebrae in your neck are susceptible to the spread of cancer or infection, as are the vertebrae in the rest of your spine. Although acute neck pain is most likely to come from a worn-out disc, in rare cases infection or spontaneous fracture may be the cause. Also, you should know that chest pain radiating into the neck from the chest could be a symptom of a heart attack.

Most acute episodes of benign back pain occur when we are in our 20s and 30s, and most of these attacks are self-limiting and are not a symptom of anything seriously wrong. Back pain tends to become more of an annoyance as we get into our 40s and 50s; the attacks are not as severe, but they may be more nagging and last longer. However, it is during these years that we most commonly suffer from disc herniations. I will tell you all about disc herniation in Chapter 5.

If you have acute lingering back pain that worries you, who should you see for it? How do you choose between the many different types of doctors and therapists? I will explore this issue in the next chapter.

CHAPTER 4

Choosing the Right Kind of Doctor

There are so many types of doctors and other health care providers who treat back pain that this entire chapter will be devoted to this subject. I also touch upon this subject in other chapters where it is appropriate to the problem, i.e., spine surgeon for surgery, pain management specialist for an epidural steroid injection, and physical therapist for pain control and improvement in strength, stamina, and balance. This chapter will be a specific description of the various specialties and services that are available to help you with your back problem.

I have seen people who have been treating their back pain by going directly to an acupuncturist or massage therapist only to find out that in doing so they delayed getting a timely diagnosis and treatment for a serious problem.

Acute, intermittent, or chronic back pain may cause us to seek medical help in various ways. We can be carried to the emergency room of our local hospital in agony, or, if our back pain allows, we make an appointment to see a doctor at some time in the future. Depending on the type of medical insurance we have, HMO, PPO, or no insurance at all, we may go to our primary care physician, to the neighborhood chiropractor, or we may refer ourselves directly to a specialist such as an orthopaedic surgeon or physical therapist. Here are descriptions of most of the types of health care providers who manage back pain syndromes and the expertise that they can provide you.

Emergency physician and acute back pain

If you seek help in an emergency room for acute back pain, the ER doctor will evaluate you to be sure you are not suffering from a serious life- or limb-threatening emergency such as cauda equina syndrome or an aneurysm (pages 30, 33). If you have a serious problem that requires admission to the hospital, they will immediately call in an appropriate specialist for your condition, i.e. a spinal surgeon for cauda equina syndrome, a urologist for a kidney stone, or a vascular surgeon for an aneurysm. If the ER doctor diagnoses you with an episode of acute back pain that is not life- or limb-threatening (idiopathic low-back pain, see page 29), he or she will then try to help you with pain medication, muscle relaxants, and/or anti-inflammatory medication and send you home with a recommendation to follow up with your primary care physician (PCP) or a specialist such as an orthopaedist.

When should I see my primary care physician for my back?

Most people who have an acute attack of back pain do not require emergency care and have time to go to a PCP to determine how to get relief. PCPs are trained in general medical diagnosis and treatment. Traditionally, PCPs are medical doctors or osteopathic doctors who are trained in general medical care but do not have specialty training (they are also called general practitioners). Family medicine specialists are medical or osteopathic physicians who take at least two additional years of training following four years of medical school and one year of internship in general medicine. General practitioners and family medicine specialists, along with internal medicine specialists (who have three additional years of residency training in general medicine), comprise the category of qualified PCPs who can determine what is causing your back pain.

Some people who are suffering from back pain go directly to a chiropractor, physical therapist, massage therapist, or acupuncturist for relief. Although their main concern is usually to obtain relief from the pain, it is actually more important for them to find out what is causing the problem first. I would advise them to go to a PCP initially, and once the PCP has determined what is wrong, ask them to prescribe initial pain-relief measures, e.g. pain medication, physical therapy, adjustments, or acupuncture. If you do not obtain relief from these initial treatments, then your PCP should refer you to the appropriate specialist. I have seen people who have been treating their back pain by going directly to an acupuncturist or massage therapist only to find out that in doing so they delayed getting a timely diagnosis and treatment for a serious problem.

Any time a child or young person under the age of 18 is suffering from spine pain you should take them to a pediatrician or to a PCP if a pediatrician is not available. Do not take them for chiropractic or physical therapy treatment before their problem has been properly diagnosed.

Your PCP should listen to your medical history, perform a physical examination, and, when appropriate, order x-rays, laboratory tests, and an MRI to help diagnose your problem. Some states license chiropractors and physical therapists to assume the role of primary caretakers for musculoskeletal conditions such as back pain. They are allowed by law in these states to perform the same diagnostic tests as PCPs to determine why you are having spine pain. I think PCPs who are trained in general medical diagnosis and treatment are better qualified to initially manage your back pain. It is not in your best interest to directly consult a chiropractor, physical therapist, pain management specialist, acupuncturist, personal trainer, or massage therapist before the actual cause of your spine pain is diagnosed. You must be sure the pain is not a warning of a serious problem that requires referral to another type of specialist, such as a vascular surgeon.

Depending on the diagnosis and severity of your back pain, your primary care provider may refer you to another specialist, such as a physiatrist for rehabilitation or a spine surgeon for surgery.

What are physiatrists, and what can they do for me?

Physiatrists are specialists in physical medicine and rehabilitation. They are diagnosticians as well as organizers and coordinators of various treatments aimed at relieving pain and restoring function. To be designated a physiatrist you must be a medical doctor or osteopathic physician and complete an accredited residency-training program in physical medicine and rehabilitation and pass certifying board examinations. The physiatrists with whom I work with in our multi-specialty spine clinic perform careful patient histories, physical examinations, order appropriate diagnostic tests, refer patients when necessary, and formulate and coordinate a plan for treatment. They perform some diagnostic tests, such as EMG (electromyography, which is a test performed with a needle electrode to evaluate certain types of muscle and nerve diseases, page 82). They are oriented toward non-operative rehabilitation treatment. They coordinate referral to other specialists, prescribe medications and physical therapy, and perform special pain-relieving procedures, such as epidural steroid injections (see page 58). When it is appropriate, they refer patients to the spinal surgeons in our group and manage their pre-operative preparation and post-surgical follow-up.

What is a spinal surgeon?

If it is determined that you are significantly impaired from a herniated disc, spinal stenosis, trauma, deformity, tumor, and/or infection of the spine, you should be referred to a spine surgeon. Spine surgery, per se, is performed exclusively by neurosurgeons and orthopaedic surgeons. The exception is that interventional radiologists and physiatrists are performing some procedures such as vertebroplasty and kyphoplasty, (injection of bone cement into collapsed vertebrae caused by osteoporosis and tumors).

In the past 20 years, most spine surgeons are fellowship trained. To be designated a fellowship-trained spine surgeon, the physician must complete special training in diagnosis and surgical treatment of spinal conditions in an accredited spine fellowship. This year or two of special training in spinal surgery usually follows four years of medical or osteopathic school and between five and seven years of specialty training in orthopaedics or neurosurgery, respectively. Specific board examinations in spine surgery or added certificates of qualification are not currently required for designation of fellowship training.

Do I need a neurosurgeon or an orthopaedic surgeon?

Orthopaedic and neurosurgical spine surgeons are cross-trained in each other's specialties with some exceptions. Orthopaedists are more oriented toward correction of spinal deformity and spinal fusion with metal fixation devices, and neurosurgeons are oriented toward the treatment of spinal cord diseases, injuries, and tumors. However, most spinal surgeons today who have been trained in a well-known spine fellowship program are qualified to perform all aspects of diagnosis and surgical treatment of spinal diseases.

Most pediatric orthopaedic surgeons have had special training in non-operative and operative treatment of scoliosis (curvature of the spine) in patients up to the age of 18. The first spinal surgery I learned how to perform in the 1960s was from a world-renowned children's scoliosis surgeon. The children's scoliosis surgeons were the ones who developed and taught all of us – orthopaedist and neurosurgeons – how to effectively correct deformity and stabilize the spine.

I was also trained by orthopaedists and neurosurgeons in spinal surgery, but no organized fellowships in spine surgery were available until the early 1980s after I had already trained. I have participated in the training of spine surgeons since that time.

I am often asked by patients to whom I have recommended spine surgery if it is necessary for a neurosurgeon to be present. Only rare, difficult, and painful spinal problems require that both a neurosurgeon and an orthopaedic spine surgeon be present at the same time for a surgical procedure. These difficult cases usually involve tumors, infections, some spinal deformities, or spinal cord diseases and require the expertise of both specialties. The vast majority of operations for painful spinal conditions, e.g. herniated discs and spinal stenosis, can be managed by a qualified spine surgeon, be they orthopaedic or neurosurgeon.

Rheumatologists, neurologists, pain management, and other specialists

Some of the other specialties that your PCP, physiatrist, or chiropractor may refer you to, depending on the problem that is causing your spine pain, include: rheumatologist, neurologist, pain management specialist, urologist, vascular surgeon, and orthopaedic joint-replacement specialist.

A rheumatologist specializes in the diagnosis and treatment of arthritis and other painful diseases of the bones, joints, and spine. I refer any patient with back pain whom I suspect of having specific types of painful arthritis of the spine such as ankylosing spondylitis (see page 101), to our rheumatologist. Painful spinal arthritis requires a lifetime of treatment with a specific supervised exercise program and anti-inflammatory medications, and is best managed by a rheumatologist working in conjunction with your PCP.

Rheumatoid arthritis, a potentially crippling form of arthritis, can dangerously involve the neck and other areas of the spine. Rheumatologists are aware of this and will frequently refer patients to spinal surgeons for consultation, and vice versa, when we see a patient who has rheumatoid arthritis involving the neck, we refer the patient to a rheumatologist for medical management.

I will occasionally see a patient who has difficulty walking because of leg pain that can be relieved by rest. When I examine them I notice that they have a shuffling gait and a tremor of their hands. I suspect that they have Parkinson's disease as well as spinal stenosis (Chapter 6). I also see patients who have numbness in their feet and lower legs, who I suspect have peripheral neuropathy (see page 113). Neurologists, who are specialists in diseases of the brain, spinal cord, and nerves, can determine which disease is causing these symptoms and whether the person has a combination of diseases. They are qualified to treat these conditions medically.

I once saw a patient who had the spontaneous onset of a foot drop (see page 49). Foot drop, or other forms of muscle weakness of the extremities caused by a spinal condition, is usually associated with pain. Since the patient had no back or leg pain, I suspected another diagnosis and referred the patient to a neurologist. He performed an EMG (see page 82) and diagnosed Lou Gehrig's disease, (amyotrophic lateral sclerosis) a progressive, disabling condition that causes progressive muscle weakness and wasting. Neurologists perform many specialized tests, including EMGs and nerve conduction velocities.

Chiropractic medicine is primarily associated with the treatment of acute back and neck pain syndromes (Chapter 9). Chiropractic is based upon a concept of joint misalignment (subluxation), particularly of the spine. Chiropractic doctors diagnose and treat back pain with a variety of methods similar to physical therapists. They include musculoskeletal evaluation, adjustments, deep massage, stretching maneuvers, heat, ultrasound, braces, and traction devices (Chapter 9). They do not perform injections or surgery on the spine.

Physical therapists are primarily trained in the assessment of musculoskeletal disabilities and the restoration of function through pain management using physical methods such as deep massage, heat and ice, as well as improvement in strength, stamina, and agility. They also use various other methods such as special stretching devices, traction systems, and electrical stimulation. In recent years, they are also assuming responsibilities for primary care of musculoskeletal conditions, including diagnosis and treatment, in some states. More will be said about the role of physical therapists in Chapter 9.

Pain management specialists are usually medical doctors who are primarily anesthesiologists. They perform special pain injection techniques, such as epidural steroid injections for herniated discs (page 58). They also manage long-term use of narcotic pain medications for chronically ill patients such as cancer patients. They usually do not participate in the diagnosis of the cause of your back pain except when they confirm the diagnosis of the site of nerve entrapment by performing local anesthesia blocks.

Massage therapists, acupuncturists, and personal trainers

Massage therapists, acupuncturists, and personal trainers are not medically trained and do not assume responsibility for diagnosis or treatment of your painful spine condition. Your doctor should advise you when and if it is safe for you to be treated by these types of specialists (Chapter 4).

On rare occasions, back pain is from a kidney problem and requires the services of a urologist, or sometimes it's a vascular problem that requires a vascular surgeon. Obstetricians and gynecologists will occasionally consult me for an opinion regarding the source of pelvic pain or whether it is safe for a woman who suffers from back pain to become pregnant. I have frequently been consulted to help a patient who suffers from back pain during pregnancy, and on very rare occasions have had to perform disc surgery on a pregnant woman (see page 47).

Your best approach to getting an accurate diagnosis and correct treatment of initial episodes of back pain is to consult a qualified PCP and have them determine what is wrong and who you should be referred to for further diagnosis and long-term treatment. Even if you are suffering from a recurrent episode of back pain after a pain-free interval, you should still go back to your PCP because the current episode may be caused by something different. It is not a good idea to have any form of treatment without first having a specific diagnosis by a qualified physician.

CHAPTER 5

What You Should Know – And Do – If You Have a Herniated ("Slipped") Disc

What is a herniated disc, how does it happen, and why is that important to know? My MRI shows a disc herniation and the doctor told me I need surgery, but the pain is going away, so do I still need the surgery? What causes spinal discs to herniate out of place?

Contrary to the popular myth, discs do not slip out of place from between the vertebrae. What really happens is that the spongy central part (nucleus pulposus) of the disc actually squeezes through ruptures in the outer rim of the disc. Recall in the first chapter how I explained the analogy between a partially flat tire and a degenerated disc. Both the flat tire and the degenerated disc are susceptible to tears in their outer rim and subsequent blowout. In the case of the disc, the spongy center substance actually squeezes through the tears in the outer rim

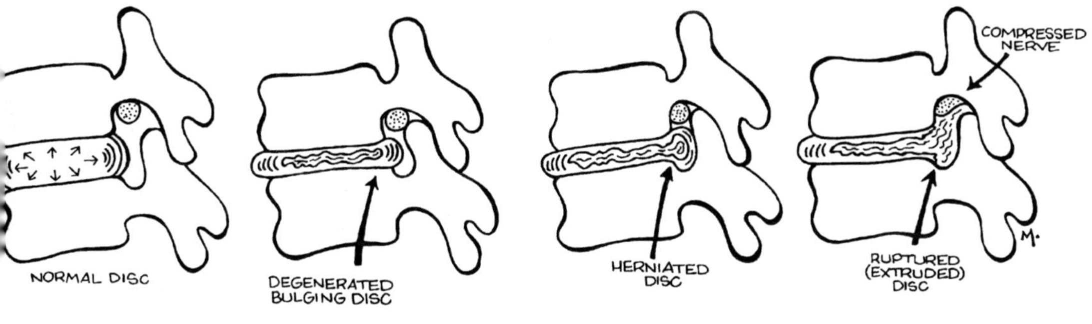

of the defective disc. This is what we call a disc herniation. There are varying degrees of disc herniation: bulging discs, prolapsed discs, extruded discs, and sequestered discs (free fragments).

Disc herniation can occur in any of the 23 discs throughout our spine and in any direction at each disc, backward toward the spinal canal and nerves, sideways, or forward. The most common level of disc herniation in humans is the lowest disc in the low back, between the fifth lumbar disc and the sacrum, the bone that attaches your spine to your pelvis. Most commonly this disc, the L5-S1 disc, herniates backward into the spinal canal and compresses the sciatic nerve, causing pain to radiate down the back of the leg from the buttocks to as far as the bottom and outside of the foot and little toes (sciatica). An L5-S1 disc herniation in your low back can result in leg pain that is worse than any toothache!

One day I received a call at work from a doctor who lived next door to one of my neighbors. My neighbor had called the doctor for help because he was experiencing severe back and leg pain. The pain was so severe that the doctor was concerned that my friend had something terrible, such as a ruptured aneurysm. On the phone I instructed the doctor to slowly lift my neighbor's painful leg to see if it made the pain worse. The doctor could only lift his leg a few inches from the bed without my neighbor screaming with pain shooting down the back of his leg. I suspected that my neighbor had a herniated disc in his low back, pressing on his sciatic nerve.

When I saw my neighbor in the emergency room, his pain was so severe he could hardly move, and after examining him I ordered an MRI scan (more about this test later in this chapter), which confirmed my suspicion that he had a herniated disc. In surgery I found that the disc herniation was pressing directly on the nerve that goes down the back of the leg to the foot. After the surgery, that same day, my neighbor was able to get out of bed by himself without leg pain. He went home the next day and was playing tennis six weeks later.

He has never forgotten how much pain his disc herniation caused or how much relief he had from the surgery, and has remained grateful for my quick diagnosis and treatment. He gave me permission to use his story in this book as an example of how painful a disc herniation can be.

Do I need surgery for my herniated disc?

One of the worst scenarios that can occur from a massive disc herniation in the low back is cauda equina syndrome (page 30). The patient goes to an emergency room in agonizing pain, only to be placed on a stretcher to wait for a doctor who is totally overwhelmed with one or more life-threatening emergencies, such as a heart attack or bleeding trauma victim. Then the pressure of the disc causes all of the nerves to the legs, bowel, and bladder to stop functioning, and the patient feels relief from the horrible pain but fails to realize that he cannot urinate and that the pelvic area is numb and the legs weak (cauda equina syndrome). The patient is indifferent to the severity of his condition because the terrible pain has gone away, so he lies quietly on the stretcher, not complaining. The doctor, exhausted from taking care of the life-threatening emergencies, glances at the patient, lying quietly on the stretcher, sees that he is no longer in pain, takes a much-needed coffee break, and later realizes the severity of the patient's problem.

Fortunately, fewer than one in 1,000 individuals who suffer from a herniated disc in the low back have cauda equina syndrome. But it can occur, and when it does, the symptoms may be ignored by the afflicted person and overlooked by those from whom they seek help. Massive disc herniation resulting in paralysis can occur, and although it is extremely rare, everyone who suffers from back pain should be aware of this possibility. If you have any of the symptoms described above, get help immediately!

Is it possible to avoid surgery for a herniated disc?

The severe pain my neighbor experienced and the massive disc herniation that leads to cauda equina syndrome are fortunately rare. *Most* people with a disc herniation suffer moderate pain that is not crippling, with or without loss of sensation, and/or mild weakness of one leg or arm. These grumbling symptoms cause deterioration in the person's quality of life but do not endanger function to the point of permanent disability.

For example, I saw a patient who was complaining of severe pain in the front of her thigh, associated with a patch of numbness and loss of sensation, and a feeling of weakness in her knee. She had been suffering with these symptoms for two months, but she said the pain had been gradually becoming less severe in the past week. An MRI scan (more about MRI shortly) showed the culprit to be a disc that had squirted into the spinal canal, pressing on a spinal nerve and causing her pain. She was taking a muscle relaxant, had been on bed rest for a few days, and was told that surgery was the only way to get relief from the pain. From my previous experience, however, I was certain that she would get better without surgery. I suggested that she stop taking the muscle relaxant that was not relieving her pain anyway. For pain control I prescribed an epidural steroid injection (more about epidurals later in this chapter). She returned to see me two weeks later, saying that she had stopped the muscle relaxant and not taken the steroid injection because the pain had subsided on its own shortly after she had seen me. She continued to improve, and the last time I saw her she was completely pain free.

The majority of patients who suffer from a disc herniation will get better spontaneously and fully recover their strength and feeling within four months of onset of the symptoms. This is because the body has defense mechanisms that dissolve the disc away. Only a few disc herniations cause intractable pain, nerve damage, paralysis, or loss of bladder and bowel function. You should not be frightened when an MRI scan indicates that you have a disc herniation unless it is causing you to have severe symptoms, such as weakness in your legs or arms, or loss of bladder and bowel function. In this case you do need surgery, and surgery can help. If you do not have such drastic symptoms, and your pain is getting better or it is not crippling, you have time to see if it will go away by itself. If the pain from a herniated disc anywhere in your spine does not go away with time (at least three months from onset) and it interferes with your quality of life, you can always have surgery later to remove that part of the disc that is pressing on your nerve (disc excision).

In my experience, the symptoms from a disc herniation rarely get worse after the initial attack. If the person is getting better after the peak of their pain, and does not have nerve damage, they rarely get worse later. It is safe for you to wait out the symptoms of a disc herniation as long as you do not have the symptoms of disabling nerve damage described above.

To further illustrate when you should have surgery for a herniated disc, I will relate the story of four pregnant patients who developed symptoms of progressive nerve damage from herniated discs and were operated upon. They all had relief of pain, recovered normal function, and had normal babies.

One of the women had severe pain, significant loss of strength in her legs, and difficulty passing urine (cauda equina syndrome) because of a herniated disc in her low back – and she was eight months pregnant. We were afraid that the strain of labor would make the disc herniate more and cause permanent paralysis. Her obstetrician delivered her normal baby by cesarean section after which, under the same anesthesia, I performed a disc excision. She was able to walk normally the same day of surgery and recovered all of her normal nerve function.

Another of the four patients had cauda equina syndrome from a massive disc herniation in her low back, and she was five months pregnant! We performed a disc excision and she delivered a normal baby at term. Five years later she and her daughter were featured on a poster for the American Academy of Orthopaedic Surgeons. They took my wife and me out to dinner to celebrate the 10th anniversary of her surgery.

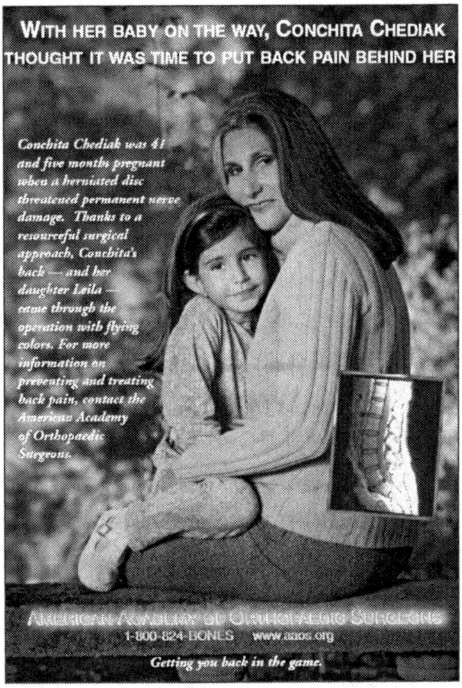

This American Academy of Orthopaedic Surgeons Poster features a patient of the author's who had cauda equina syndrome from a massive disc herniation during pregnancy. It was successfully treated with surgery.

The other two patients had similar stories and outcomes. Both had weakness in major muscles of their legs and loss of sensation from herniated discs in their backs. Both patients had complete recovery of nerve function, relief of pain, and delivered normal babies at term. The point is that if you need surgery for a herniated disc, you need it! And the results can be excellent even if you are pregnant.

How could I have a herniated disc? I wasn't injured.

Another myth is that disc herniation is the result of trauma. The truth is that normal discs do not herniate. In fact, the discs are so tough that the adjacent vertebrae will break as the result of a fall but the nearby discs will not rupture. There must be some deterioration in the disc (degeneration) for the disc to displace or herniate from the normal position between the vertebrae. Simply bending over is all it takes to herniate a degenerated disc when it is ready to fail, much like the potential for a rotting tree to blow over in a mild windstorm (the straw that broke the camel's back analogy). That is why it is so confusing for people who suffer from a painful disc herniation. They often cannot remember what brought on the pain!

Unlike in adults, trauma *can* cause normal discs to herniate in growing children. Children under the age of 16 have a growth plate on their vertebrae at the point where the strongest attachment of the disc to the vertebrae occurs. A separation of this growth plate can occur as the result of trauma, causing the disc to herniate even though it is perfectly normal otherwise. The youngest patient I ever operated upon for a disc herniation, a 12-year-old, had such an injury to a normal disc as the result of a fall from a jungle gym. Back pain in children, be it from injury or otherwise, should be considered serious and requires medical attention.

Some people have a strong genetic disposition to disc herniation. One of my 25-year-old orthopaedic residents was assisting me in surgery when he experienced a sudden onset of pain shooting down his leg from his back. "It's happened again!" he said. "I have another herniated disc." And sure enough he did, at the L5-S1. At the age of 16 he had undergone a disc excision for a herniated disc at the L3-4 level in his low back. At the age of 21 he had surgery for a L4-5 disc herniation. I removed his L5-S1 disc herniation and he returned to work within a week of surgery. He subsequently became an accomplished surgeon. He was in excellent physical condition when I operated on him, and remains that way, swimming a mile a day to stay in shape. He has a busy practice and a good quality of life despite a strong genetic predisposition to herniate discs.

What are the symptoms of a herniated disc?

Most herniated discs produce pain in one leg or one arm. Less commonly a disc will cause only back pain or pain in both legs and both arms. The pain associated with a disc herniation usually radiates from the back down the leg, the neck down the arm, or from the back of the chest to the front along the ribs, depending on the site of the herniation. The pain is described as any combination of the following sensations: burning, numbness, pins and needles, aching, and stabbing. Most people describe attacks of neck or back pain leading up to the pain that radiates into the arm or leg. The pain may be associated with loss of sensation and/or weakness of handgrip from a disc herniation in the neck and an inability to lift the foot (foot drop) from a disc herniation in the low back.

I always have my patients fill out a pain drawing so that I can immediately tell the location and characteristics of the pain. When I first see a patient's self-generated pain drawing, I not only can tell that they have a herniated disc, but I can also tell you which nerve it is pressing on. For example, a patient with an L5-S1 disc herniation in the low back pressing on the first sacral nerve root will place symbols depicting pain down the back of the thigh, lower leg, and into the bottom and side of the foot. The symbols on the pain drawing may designate any combination of abnormal sensations such as stabbing pain, burning, numbness, tingling, and aching.

A herniated disc in the low back may cause you to lean over like the Tower of Pisa and to have a painful limp. A disc in the neck can cause you to stumble and trip and lose your balance (my aunt's symptoms). A disc in the low back can cause inability to urinate or constipation. If you experience gait disturbance or change in bowel and bladder function associated with spine pain, notify your doctor immediately. If your pain lasts for more than a few days, interferes with your sleep, or requires that you take pain medication, you need to see your doctor to determine what is wrong.

To diagnose a disc herniation, your doctor will listen to you describe your symptoms and then perform a physical examination. Your doctor

Please fill out the pain drawing. This will tell us where your pain is now and something about it.

Using the appropriate symbol mark the areas on your body where you feel the pain.

-- Numbness 000 Pins & Needles xxx Burning +++ Aching
/// Stabbing *** Other ☐ No Pain

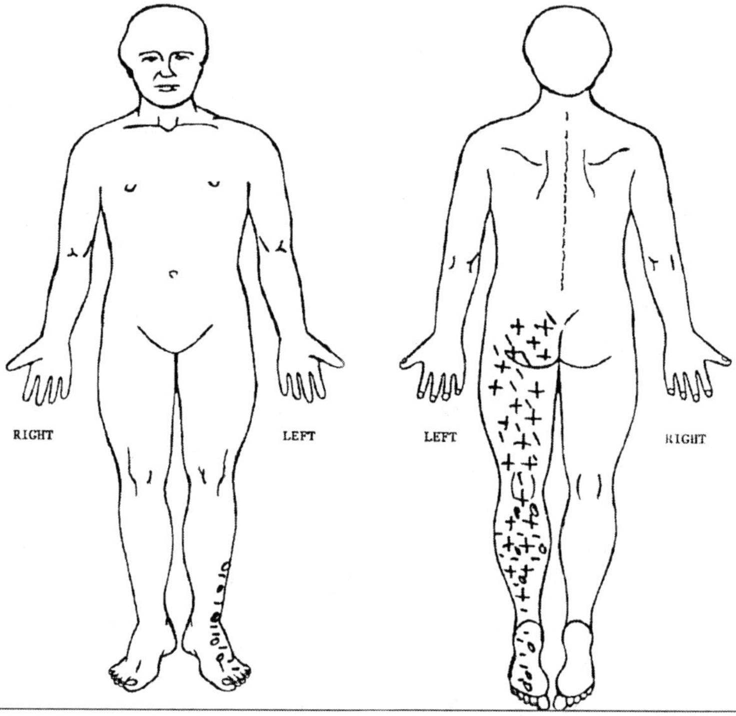

This patient-generated pain drawing depicts typical left sciatic leg pain from a herniated disc between the 5th lumbar vertebra and the sacrum (L5-S1 HNP).

will have you walk on your toes and on your heels to check your strength and coordination; look at your spine to see if it is straight or leaning to one side and have you bend forward as far as the pain allows to determine if you have muscle spasm; check to see if you have lost any reflexes or if you have abnormal reflexes (I discovered abnormal reflexes when I examined my aunt, which told me she had something seriously wrong); determine if you have lost any sensation or muscle strength; and check to see that you have good circulation in your legs, arms, and neck.

There are a few maneuvers that will stretch the nerve over a disc herniation and reproduce the pain that you have to confirm that diagnosis. One test that is specific for detecting a disc herniation in the low back is the so-called straight-leg-raising test. While you are lying on your back facing up, the doctor slowly raises the painful leg while keeping your knee straight. The degree of elevation of the leg from the table and the degree of reproduction of the pain radiating down your leg is an indication of how much the disc is pressing on the nerve in your back. I could only lift my neighbor's painful leg a few degrees before he screamed from the pain all the way from his back, down the leg, and to his foot. Even more ominous was that when I lifted his opposite leg, the pain was reproduced in his painful leg; this is called the crossed-straight-leg-raising test. The tests told me that the disc had squeezed completely into the spinal canal and that is exactly where I found it at surgery.

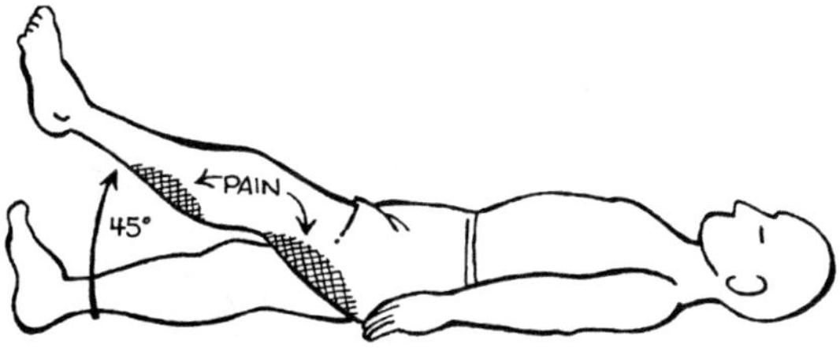

STRAIGHT-LEG-RAISING TEST

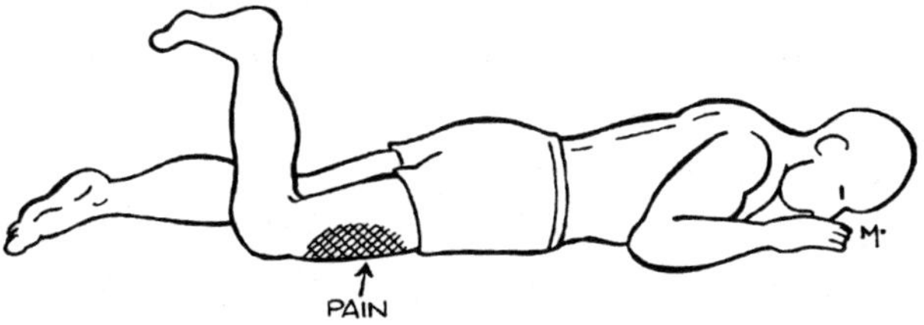

FEMORAL-STRETCH TEST

Warning: If you are having severe pain in your arm or leg, do not have someone other than a doctor try these tests on you, because it may make the pain even worse! When the doctor goes to perform the tests, tell her or him to go slowly and stop as soon as you feel the pain get worse. When I was a resident in training I unknowingly lifted a colleague's leg too fast and too far, which exacerbated his leg pain so much that he could not sleep that night. The test did confirm my suspicion that he had a herniated disc in his low back, but he wouldn't talk to me after that, and he insisted that someone else take care of him.

There are two other variations of the nerve-root-tension test. The first is the femoral-stretch test (see the illustration on this page), in which you lie face down and the doctor bends your knee. If you experience pain in the front of your thigh, it may mean that you have a disc herniation in the upper part of your low back (the L2-3, L3-4, or L4-5 disc). The second variation is the straight-arm-raising test where the doctor raises your arm sideways and backward. Reproduction of arm pain with this maneuver may mean that you have a disc herniation in your neck (most common levels are C5-6 and C6-7).

How does an MRI scan work, and how can it tell me I have a herniated disc? And what is a CAT scan and a myelogram?

After hearing your story and examining you, the most accurate, safest, least painful, and most cost-effective test your doctor can order to confirm the diagnosis of a disc herniation is an MRI scan. The MRI scan has replaced the myelogram and CAT scan for diagnosis of herniated discs and most other spinal disorders. For this reason I will describe what this test is, how it works, how it is performed and what it shows.

When I started in practice, we would confirm the diagnosis of a disc herniation by performing a myelogram, a painful procedure that involved inserting a needle into the spinal canal, injecting a painful oily dye, and taking numerous x-rays. The disc would appear as an indentation on the dye column. The test was painful, required hospitalization and x-ray exposure, and could be dangerous. Later the CAT scan, a three-dimensional x-ray, was developed. It could detect a herniated disc without performing a myelogram, but the patient was still exposed to x-rays, and the pictures from a CAT scan were not very clear. Then new water-soluble myelogram dyes were developed that weren't as painful or potentially harmful as the older oil-based dyes, and they could be used with the CAT scans to make them more accurate. This method is still used to diagnose spinal conditions in patients who cannot have an MRI scan, such as those with metal implants near the spine and people with heart pacemakers.

In the early 1980s the MRI scan was developed for diagnosis. This procedure was a dramatic development in all of medicine but was especially beneficial for the diagnosis of painful spinal disorders. It is a painless procedure, safe – even during pregnancy (no x-ray exposure) – and extremely accurate. MRI scans are the only way to determine exactly where and how far the disc has herniated into the spinal canal (see MRI scan this page). The picture of the spine produced by an MRI is so accurate that it can provide the surgeon with an exact map as to where to find a herniated disc fragment in the spinal canal.

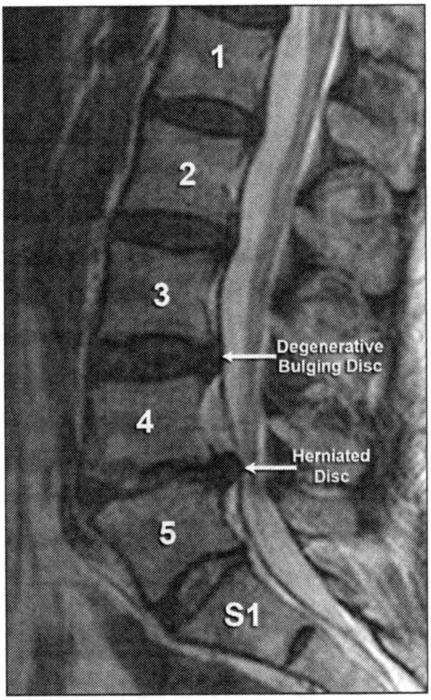

This side-view MRI scan of the low back shows a herniated disc between the 4th and 5th lumbar vertebrae and a bulging disc between the 3rd and 4th vertebrae.).

MRI stands for magnetic resonance imaging. In order to understand how it works, recall when you were in science class learning about how a magnet works. When you place a magnet under a paper containing iron filings, the little pieces of iron arrange themselves on the paper in the orientation of the magnetic field of the magnet. If you rotate the magnet under the paper, the iron filings re-distribute themselves to align to the new orientation of the magnetic field. Picture all of the trillions of water molecules in your body as iron filings, and place them in a magnetic field that is made to oscillate back and forth. The water molecules will orient themselves first one way and then another and begin to wobble. Given a few trillion molecules wobbling all in the same direction, they give off a signal, resonance, which can be detected and converted into a picture by a computer. The water molecules in your body will resonate differently according to where they are located in your body, such as in discs, spinal fluid, fat, bone, or muscle. MRI scanners are comprised of large magnets to make the water molecules in your body resonate, and computers that can detect the resonance and produce a clear picture of parts of your body such as the discs in your back.

Using an MRI scan, your doctor can distinguish different tissues in your body such as disc, bone, fat, muscle, blood, spinal fluid, scar tissue, and ligaments. It can distinguish normal from degenerated and herniated discs. You can see the degree to which a disc is degenerated on an MRI scan. The scan can tell you how far out into the canal a disc has herniated. Tumors, infections, and fractures can be detected by MRI scans.

No other diagnostic test can provide you with so much information concerning what is wrong in your back. And yet MRI scans are safe, accurate, cost-effective, create no x-ray exposure, and can be performed on almost everyone except patients who have metal implants in the exact area of their spine that must be seen. Stainless steel screws and rods in the spine will interfere with the MRI scan picture. People with a heart pacemaker should not have an MRI scan (magnetic fields can interfere with the function of a pacemaker). People who have some other magnetic metal foreign objects in their body should not have MRI scans. However, you can have an MRI if you have a metal joint replacement in your hip, knee, shoulder, or ankle. Also, most metal bone plates, rods, and screws for fracture fixation are compatible with having an MRI scan. Spine implants made of titanium steel do not interfere with the MRI scan as much as stainless-steel implants. People with a stainless-steel implant in their spine or who have a heart pacemaker should have a CAT scan and/or a myelogram instead of an MRI to diagnose their problem.

What is it like to have an MRI scan, and what do I do if I am claustrophobic?

When the first MRI scan arrived in our clinic in the early 1980s, I volunteered to have one performed on me, in order to understand what my patients would experience and to be able to advise them about the study. I was also curious to find out if an MRI scan could tell me why I had suffered from periodic bouts of back pain. I was placed face-up on a thin stretcher on tracks and was slid into a tunnel in the scanner that was about 10 feet long and open at both ends. My face was less than a foot from the wall of the tunnel. As the scan began there was a loud, incessant thumping noise; I surmised this was the magnetic field being shifted back and forth. After a short period of time I became very anxious, my heart began to beat fast, and I started to breathe heavily. I felt afraid and shouted, "Get me out of here!" It seemed like an eternity, although it was probably only a few seconds, before they pulled me out of the scanner. I had suffered from a claustrophobic attack. I never had any clue before that time that I had claustrophobia (irrational fear of small, enclosed spaces). As a result of my claustrophobic experience in the MRI scanner, I developed some ways to prevent this from happening to others. I will pass them on to you.

Why not an open scanner if I am claustrophobic?

Open MRI scans have been developed for the claustrophobic patient. Unfortunately, the pictures produced by the open scanners are not as clear and accurate as those from the closed scanners. I often see patients who come to my clinic with an MRI scan that was performed in an open scanner, and the scan is usually inadequate to clearly localize the cause of their pain. The patient ends up needing to have another scan performed in a closed scanner in order to make the diagnosis, much to their distress and to that of their insurance company.

To get the claustrophobic patient through a closed MRI scan without a reaction, I suggest the following measures. I first explain the importance of using a closed scanner to accurately diagnose their problem and the inadequacy of an open scanner for this purpose. I tell my patients to tell the technician who is performing the scan about their claustrophobia and that they want to be removed from the scanner at the first sign they become anxious. I recommend that they have a relative or friend drive them to the MRI facility and sit with them through the scan. Finally, I prescribe a sedative to be taken just before the scan. Using these measures, I was personally able to have an MRI scan of my spine several years after my first unsuccessful attempt. These measures and advice have proven to be very helpful for my claustrophobic patients who would not otherwise have been able to obtain an MRI scan. Even if you are claustrophobic, these recommendations should help you to successfully obtain an accurate MRI scan.

The picture of the spine obtained from a good MRI so clearly shows the reason for the pain that it is easy for my patients to see the problem when I show it to them (see page 53). The only problem with the MRI is that it sometimes shows too much information. A famous spinal surgeon and mentor once told me that the doctor who treats the image on the x-ray is a shadow boxer, and the doctor who treats the patient is a heavyweight. This means that the indication for surgery is not the appearance of a herniated disc in the patient's MRI scan, but the patient's pain and disability resulting from the disc herniation. The patient's symptoms and disability must be confirmed by the MRI scan for the test to be useful. Many a time I have seen a disc herniation in an MRI scan that is on the side opposite of the patient's pain. After further scrutiny the real culprit producing the pain becomes apparent on the correct side, and the disc on the non-painful side is of no consequence. We know from our discussion in the first chapter of this book that not all disc herniations produce pain. I have seen patients who were told they needed surgery because of a large disc herniation that was seen on their MRI. The patient seeks another opinion because their pain is not so bad, and they instinctively know that surgery is not completely necessary. I reassure them that they can safely avoid surgery and that they will eventually get better with time despite the appearance of a large disc herniation on their MRI scan.

What can I do to avoid surgery for my herniated disc?

You have been told that you have a herniated disc on your MRI scan and that you need surgery, but you are getting around all right and you do not have severe pain, weakness, or loss of bowel and bladder function forcing you to have emergency surgery. What are your options? Most people with disc herniations fall into this category. They can get around, but that is about it. Something must be done so that they can sleep, go to work, and eventually get back to normal.

First of all, it has been proven that if you can live through the pain without surgery, you have better than an 80 percent chance of full recovery (no pain, full function, no nerve damage) within one year and 92 percent in 10 years. This is the same chance of recovery that you can expect with surgery! It seems obvious that waiting is safer than having surgery. But that is not necessarily true if you develop a complication from non-operative treatment, such as becoming habituated to pain medications, developing a bleeding ulcer from anti-inflammatory medication, or developing an infection from an injection. So then what is the safest and most effective course of action: surgery or no surgery?

I advise my patients who have a painful disc herniation that they have three options. The first is to walk it off and be as active as you can be within the limits of the pain. I reassure them that there is a good chance the disc will shrink by itself, given enough time, and that the pain will go away within four months of onset. Our bodies have normal defense mechanisms that allow this to happen. If their pain is not interfering with their sleep and work, they usually take this option. After such discussions, many a patient has told me that understanding the problem was half the cure. Knowledge of the natural history of disc herniation gave them the reassurance they needed to discontinue medical care and walk it off!

If they require pain relief in order to sleep and function, I recommend a series of one to three epidural steroid injections (I will explain what epidurals are in a moment). Epidurals are very effective in relieving pain from a herniated disc. Pain relief allows you to walk off the symptoms and keeps you from taking narcotics and muscle relaxants (commonly prescribed pain relievers), which are habit-forming, make you drowsy, and cause depression (more about this in Chapter 8 on chronic back pain). If the pain from a herniated disc is still significantly impairing their quality of life after three months of waiting for it to go away, then I recommend the third option, surgery.

Here is a further explanation for the three options in treating a painful herniated disc: walk it off, epidural steroid injection, and surgery.

What does it mean to "walk it off?"

We know from several classic studies that the natural history of symptoms from disc herniation is spontaneous resolution, if given enough time. As long as the disc has not caused progressive or severe nerve damage, it is better to try to walk the symptoms off. The secret is not to allow the pain to make you physically debilitated or mentally ill.

First you should consult a spinal specialist (see Chapter 4) who is familiar with disc problems and who should determine that your symptoms are really the result of a herniated disc.

Second, you should do only what is necessary to obtain enough pain relief so that you can get a night's sleep and get around enough to take care of yourself. This means taking as few narcotic painkillers and anti-inflammatory medications as possible. Try not to take any muscle relaxants at all, which cause too many side effects, such as drowsiness and depression. Avoid traction, hanging upside down, manipulation, and especially passive stretching of the painful extremity. Remember how I made an enemy of a colleague by performing a straight-leg-raising test? Very light massage, heat and/or ice packs – well padded so as not to burn your skin – are good for pain relief. Most of these touch measures, as well as acupuncture, will relieve pain as long as you are not taking narcotic pain medications. I will explain the reason for this in the chapter on chronic pain. Try to remain as active as possible within the limits of your pain and stamina. Walking, aquatic exercises, stationary bicycle, and treadmill aerobics all help to keep you from becoming deconditioned (out of shape). Do *not* take pain medication so that you can exercise. Remember that the pain is a warning that something is wrong, and it is a normal defense mechanism. If, because of the pain, you cannot remain active despite these measures, then you should consider the following options for your disc herniation.

What is an epidural, how does it work, and is it painful?

Epidural steroid injection (epidural) is a method of injecting a small amount of local anesthetic and steroid medication (the most powerful anti-inflammatory drug available) directly into the area of your spine where the nerve is being irritated by the herniated disc. The object is to place the potent steroid where it will do the most good. The local anesthetic is added to the injection to give you immediate pain relief and to confirm that the injection is at the correct location. Herniated discs can be a triple whammy to the nerve because they not only compress and stretch the nerve, but they leak irritants to the nerve. Epidural steroid injections are meant to block the irritants and reduce the pain. I prescribe them so that patients can get enough pain relief to avoid taking narcotic painkillers and so that they can get a good night's sleep. One of the benefits of epidural injections is that only small doses of steroids are required to be effective.

I am not an advocate of giving steroids by mouth, the so-called "dose-pacs," because it requires very high doses to get enough steroids to the area of the irritated nerve to be effective. The high doses of oral steroids required to be effective can cause some rare but harmful side effects, such as an increase in blood sugar (diabetes), loss of bone mass (osteoporosis), bleeding ulcer in your stomach, and destruction of the hip joint (aseptic necrosis of the hip). These bad side effects from steroids taken by mouth are not as common when they are given by epidural injection.

A specialist should perform the epidural injection using fluoroscopy (moving x-ray picture) to accurately place the steroid in the exact region of the painful nerve. I refer my patients to another specialist (anesthesiologist or physiatrist) to perform epidural injections. Your doctor may perform the epidural or may refer you to another specialist to have it performed.

What should I expect when I have an epidural?

First, a disclaimer: Unlike an MRI scan, I have personally never had an epidural, therefore I am relating to you what patients have told me about their experience with the procedure. Most patients say that it is not a very painful procedure, but a few patients do complain of experiencing a temporary increase in pain at the time of the injection. This is particularly true when the steroid is injected into the area of an irritated nerve. You can request sedation when it is being performed, but some patients do not want it. The injection includes a local anesthetic along with the steroid medication, which should give you some immediate pain relief. Immediate pain relief from the local anesthetic is an indication that the correct area was injected. I write a prescription stating the exact level and side of the herniated disc so that the doctor who is performing the procedure will know exactly where I want the injection to be placed. Accurate placement of the steroid is confirmed when the patient has immediate relief of pain from the local anesthetic in the injection. Immediate relief of your pain at the time of the epidural injection also helps to confirm the diagnosis that the disc herniation seen on your MRI scan is the actual cause of your pain.

What are the possible side effects from an epidural?

Diabetic patients may see a temporary increase in their blood sugar following an epidural. They should monitor their blood sugar closely for a few days following the injection. However, I have not seen a diabetic patient develop any permanent trouble from the transient elevation of blood sugar following an epidural.

Rarely, a patient may experience a spinal headache. A spinal headache results from leakage of spinal fluid when the needle causes a hole in the sac (dura) that contains the nerves. Years ago I had a spinal headache following spinal anesthesia for knee surgery. I experienced intense pain behind my eyes when I stood up and it went away immediately when I lay down. This is typically how patients describe a spinal headache. It usually goes away after a few days, but it can be very disturbing to say the least. At times a blood patch is required to stop the leak and relieve the headache (blood is taken from a vein in your arm and then injected into the epidural space to seal the spinal fluid leak). Spinal headache from spinal fluid leakage is seen more often in patients who have had more than three epidural injections. This is one of the reasons I limit the number of epidurals I will prescribe to my patients to three in a six-month period. The other reason for limiting the number of epidural steroid injections is that if three injections that lessen local inflammation do not give lasting relief of pain, then the irritating source of the problem is not being taken care of. So, if the nerve in your back continues to be irritated and painful despite three epidurals within a six-month period, then it is time to consider other options, such as surgery.

In over 35 years of practice, I have seen only two patients who developed an infection following an epidural steroid injection. Both patients were heavy smokers; smokers are susceptible to infection, so I ask my patients to stop smoking before they have an epidural. The risk of infection from an epidural is very low. In order to prevent this complication, I do not recommend that a patient with an active infection, such as acne around the site of injection, have an epidural steroid injection until the infection is treated first. If you have had a recent urinary tract infection, fever, earache, toothache, periodontal disease, foot ulcer, or other source of infection in your body, you should not have an epidural. Active infections somewhere in your body must be treated before having an epidural steroid injection because of the risk of the infection spreading to your spine as the result of the procedure. You should warn your doctor of any active or recent infections that you have experienced, even a common cold, before allowing yourself to have an epidural steroid injection.

Increased nerve damage may result from an epidural injection if the needle penetrates the nerve. A skillful doctor who performs the injection will take precautions while performing the procedure to prevent this from happening.

When appropriate precautions are taken, I have found that epidural steroid injections are a safe and effective way of relieving pain caused by a herniated disc. Many of my patients have been satisfied with the pain relief experienced from an epidural steroid for a painful herniated disc.

Band-aid surgery, micro-surgery, laminectomy: Which is best for me?

If your disc herniation causes weakness of a major muscle in your arm or leg along with the pain, if you have changes in your bowel and bladder function, or if you experience loss of balance, you need surgery as soon as possible. If the pain is unrelenting and you are having difficulty walking and sleeping, you should have surgery. If you have had the pain for more than three months and it has not been relieved by one or more epidural steroid injections and you need narcotics to function, you should seriously consider surgery.

The standard surgical procedure for a disc herniation in your

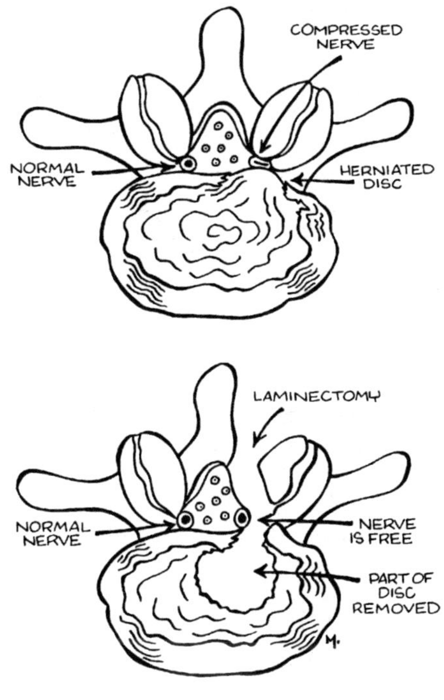

The top figure illustrates a spine cross section showing a compressed nerve from a herniated disc. The lower figure shows that a portion of the disc has been removed to decompress the nerve.

low back is called a laminectomy (removing part of the roof of the spinal canal in order to see the herniated disc) and disc excision (removing that part of the disc that is pressing on the nerve). The incision is between two and four inches long, depending on how large you are, and the surgeon wears magnifying glasses to perform the procedure. The procedure takes between 45 minutes and an hour and a half, depending on how adherent the herniated disc is to the nerve. Most patients are able to walk the same day of surgery and leave the hospital the following day. You can expect to be able to get out of bed by yourself and walk without pain before you leave the hospital. The procedure is not very painful, and most of my patients take narcotics for no more than a day or two following surgery. You can expect to be back at work within 10 days.

I once removed a herniated disc in the low back on a bone fisherman. Bone fishermen are the ones who stand on an elevated platform in the back of a skiff and push the boat through the water with a long pole. The surgery was on a Monday, and he returned to the Florida Keys the following morning. He never came back to see me in the clinic, so I contacted his wife and she told me that he was out fishing and had been since two days following his surgery! It was bone fishing season and he wasn't going to miss any more time than was necessary. He was pushing his boat with his clients around the saltwater flats of the Florida Keys in hot pursuit of bonefish.

Though I would not advocate that you try to do what he did two days following disc surgery, this story illustrates that recovery from a standard open disc excision in the low back can be that fast. My doctor colleagues have gone back to work within a week of disc surgery. But for someone who performs heavy work requiring lifting and bending, I do not recommend returning to work until six weeks following the surgery. I do not recommend golf or tennis, both of which require twisting – a particularly stressful motion for a degenerated disc – for a period of three months following a disc excision. I recommend walking exercises for the first six weeks following surgery. I have found that most people can return to the activity level they were at prior to suffering from the herniated disc. A tennis player should be able to resume playing tennis, and a golfer should be able to golf following disc surgery.

What about micro-discectomy? What is it and does it have any advantage over a standard discectomy? Micro-discectomy is the removal of the disc through a small incision (less than two inches) with the aid of a microscope. It requires more time to perform the surgery through a small surgical incision compared to a standard surgical incision. I can see no real advantage, other than cosmetic, to have the surgery performed through a small incision. The proponents of the smaller incision claim that patients leave the hospital sooner and require less pain medication following micro-discectomy compared to a standard disc excision. This has not been my observation. Patients who have a standard incision versus a micro disc incision both leave the hospital within 23 hours and are back to work within 10 days. I do not recommend the microscopic procedure to my patients unless they specifically ask for the procedure. The length of time spent in the hospital and the amount of pain medication required following surgery, including discectomy, is related to the health and fitness of the patient, not the length of the skin incision.

I saw an advertisement in a flight magazine with three ladies lying on a beach; one had a band-aid on her back from surgery the same day! How about band-aid surgery? Band-aid surgery refers to a technique in which a scope is used to remove the disc, similar to the well-known arthroscopic surgery for the knee. The incision for the scope is presumably small enough to be covered by a band-aid, albeit a large one! Over many years I have seen many failed attempts to perfect arthroscopic surgery for the spine. The method has not gained acceptance by most spinal surgeons for several reasons. The most common disc that herniates is the L5-S1 disc, which is a difficult level in the low back to safely reach through a scope. The second reason is that almost every disc herniation that doesn't get better with time is associated with a small, misshapen spine canal, spinal stenosis, which is difficult to correct through a scope. I have also seen some serious complications from this technique. There is a higher incidence of spinal-fluid leakage, infections, and nerve damage using this technique compared to standard disc surgery. I do not recommend or perform arthroscopic disc surgery for these reasons.

When they remove the disc, what do they put in its place?

Only that part of the disc that is out of place is removed in the low back, and a spinal fusion (page 93) is hardly ever performed at the same time. The discs in the low back are eight to 10 times larger than the discs in your neck, and only a small part of the discs in your low back herniates out of place. The remainder of the disc is still adequate to function normally with rare exceptions, which I will explain to you in the chapters on spinal fusion and disc replacements.

Your neck discs are small, and the area of the disc that herniates can be difficult to reach because your spinal cord is in the way. Therefore, most herniated discs in the neck are taken out by a front approach to the spine. Almost the entire disc in your neck must be removed to reach the displaced fragment in front of the spinal cord. Therefore a spinal fusion with a block of bone from your pelvis or from a bone bank is used to fill the space between the vertebrae following a disc excision in the neck. The other alternative is to have an artificial disc replacement instead of a fusion following a neck-disc removal. I will explain the pros and cons of both procedures in depth in Chapter 12.

Some disc herniations in the neck can be removed through a small incision in the back of your neck. When the procedure can be performed from this approach, a spinal fusion is not necessary because the whole disc is not removed, only the fragment that is pressing on the nerve. This is a good alternative approach to the standard front approach, which requires that the entire disc be removed and that something be put into its place.

Disc herniations in the thoracic spine, or back of the chest area, are the rarest, and they are the most difficult and dangerous to remove of any of the discs in your spine. There are two ways to remove a disc from the thoracic spine; one is from behind, just alongside the spine, and the more common way, and I think the safer way, is through the chest. This is one area of your spine where some discs can be safely taken out through a scope. Most of the disc is taken out, and a fusion is usually performed at the same time. Because there is very little normal motion in thoracic discs, unlike the neck, artificial discs are not used following the removal of a thoracic disc.

In the long run, which is better: waiting it out or having surgery?

What are the benefits of having a disc removed if it is not an emergency, and is it okay to wait? If you are faced with chronic disc pain that is not threatening life or limb and for whatever reason need to have quick relief, then there is an advantage to having a disc excision. You can expect at least 80 percent relief of pain almost immediately upon awakening from anesthesia. You may experience immediate partial relief of muscle weakness and improvement in sensory loss following a disc excision. According to studies reported in the medical literature, more people are happier the first year following surgery compared to people who wait it out. The studies also show that somewhere between the first year and 10 years following onset of the symptoms of a low-back disc herniation, the people who wait it out have the same overall relief as those who have surgery. Why have the surgery then? Many people cannot wait it out for various reasons. My neighbor had such severe pain that he wanted immediate surgery. The bone fisherman needed quick relief from his disc herniation so that he would lose as little time as possible from fishing season. Others have reached a plateau and have gotten better with time, and some patients who are gradually getting worse elect surgery. After learning from your doctor the alternatives, nature, benefits, and risks of disc surgery, you need to make the final decision about whether the surgery is right for you

What are the risks of disc surgery?

What are the risks of disc surgery in your low back? How can you avoid the risks of disc surgery? In obtaining an informed consent for surgery from my patients, I always list these risks: death, paralysis, infection, nerve damage, and spinal-fluid leakage. I go on to explain that the risk of death from anesthesia is less than one in 15,000. It is much lower in people who are in good health. Smokers are at the greatest risk for this complication, which would stem from a stroke or heart attack. You should stop smoking before having surgery and be cleared for surgery by your PCP to avoid this complication.

Many years ago there was a famous movie actor who bled to death while undergoing disc surgery as the result of the surgeon pushing an instrument through the disc into a major blood vessel in front of his spine. This is an extremely rare complication of low-back surgery. The best way to avoid this complication is to pick a well-qualified and experienced spinal surgeon – orthopaedic or neurosurgical specialist – to perform the operation. This is a dreaded complication that well-trained spine surgeons are always on the alert to avoid.

The risk of paralysis from a disc excision in the low back is less than one in 5,000. The risk of paralysis from the surgery itself is rare; it is in the day or two following surgery that bleeding in the wound can press on the nerves and cause weakness leading to paralysis (epidural hematoma). One way to prevent this complication is to stop taking anti-inflammatory medication, aspirin, vitamin E, garlic, herbal medicines, and blood thinners prior to surgery. If you have a tendency to bleed or bruise easily, you should alert your surgeon so that they can test your blood to see if it clots normally. Your doctor must take you off of Coumadin, Plavix, and other blood thinners (anti-coagulants) before having spine surgery of any kind to avoid the complication of excessive bleeding and post-operative epidural hematoma. The risks of stopping blood thinners for a period of four to six weeks around the time of spine surgery should be explained to you by the doctor who prescribed them. That doctor should be the one who coordinates with your spine surgeon about taking you off the blood thinners and putting you back on them at a specified time following the surgery.

The risk of infection from disc surgery is less than one in 100 cases. Optimizing your health prior to surgery – no smoking: smokers are 10 times more apt to have a post-operative infection compared to non-smokers – can decrease the risk of infection considerably. You should alert your surgeon if you are prone to urinary tract infections, even if you do not have symptoms at the time. Also tell your surgeon if you have a toothache, periodontal disease, earache, ulceration, or boil on your skin. If you have a cold, flu, or upper respiratory tract infection you should delay surgery. Active skin acne in the area where the incision will be made must be treated before having surgery on your spine. All of these precautions decrease the possibility of a post-operative infection following disc excision.

Nerve damage can result from surgically manipulating the already compressed nerve. Sometimes a disc fragment is stuck so tightly to the nerve that it is difficult to remove it without further stretching the nerve. When weakness or numbness occurs from this type of surgical manipulation, it will usually clear up within a few weeks of surgery. This is one reason why I think it is safer to have a routine laminectomy through an adequately sized skin incision. The surgeon can see the nerve more easily and can manipulate it more gently through this approach, thus avoiding this complication.

No matter how carefully the surgery is performed, 5 percent of the time a hole is made in the dura, the sac that contains the spinal nerves and spinal fluid. Sometimes holes are already there from a previous epidural steroid injection. Either way, they should be closed with stitches. When a hole occurs in the dura during surgery, instead of getting out of bed the night of surgery you should stay flat in bed for a day or two until the leak is sealed. Except for the dangers of bed rest and the nuisance of a spinal headache, there are usually no bad consequences from a hole in the dura. Despite these risks of disc surgery, it is a relatively safe procedure – safer than having your gall bladder removed.

There are some specific complications associated with removing a disc in the neck. The spinal cord takes up more space and is at more risk for injury in your cervical spine. Thus, spinal-cord injury with paralysis is a potential – though rare – complication of cervical-disc surgery. While surgically exposing the disc in your neck, it is possible that the nerve to your vocal cords can be stretched, causing a hoarse voice. The tube leading from your mouth to your stomach, the esophagus, can be punctured. The major vessels to and from your brain can be damaged, leading to a stroke, blindness, or death. Major things can go wrong! To avoid having one of these complications of disc surgery in your neck, choose a well-trained spinal surgeon who is experienced in neck surgery.

Disc herniations in the thoracic spine are sometimes very difficult to remove because they tend to stick tightly to the spinal cord. Some of these disc herniations are gradually causing paralysis and must be removed in an attempt to prevent this from happening. I have seen patients become paralyzed from attempts to remove these discs even by very experienced and careful surgeons. In light of these rare cases, both the patient and the doctor must have a clear understanding of the dangerous risk of paralysis, and the patient must be the one to make the final decision for surgery.

How can I avoid the risks of spine surgery?

You should consider all of the benefits and possible risks of any elective surgery (elective surgery is one that can be planned ahead of time) before having it performed. Your surgeon should discuss these issues with you, answer all of your questions, and let you make the final decision. One of the best ways to prevent bad things from happening to you, as I mentioned before, is to pick a qualified surgeon. Ask around to see if others in your community have heard of or used the surgeon and whether they have a good reputation.

My doctor is an orthopaedic spine surgeon. Do I need a neurosurgeon?

Neurosurgeons and orthopaedic surgeons specialize in spine surgery and both are fully qualified to perform a disc surgery at any level of the spine. Both specialties are trained to do most spinal surgery. Tumors involving the spinal cord and nerves are usually handled by neurosurgeons, and instrumented spinal fusions and deformity are attended to by orthopaedic surgeons. In our institution at the University of Miami Miller School of Medicine, orthopaedic and neurosurgical spine specialists work together in difficult cases involving tumors and sophisticated reconstruction of the spine that require instrumented spinal fusions. We train our residents and spine fellows together. Both specialties are fully qualified to perform most spinal surgery. This is the case in most major spine-surgery centers.

Assuming responsibility for your own health is as important as picking the right surgeon. Tell the doctor about all your medical conditions, medications, tendency to bleed, and of any recent infections; stop smoking, stop taking aspirin and other anti-inflammatories, and stop all herbal medications; lose weight if you are overweight. Overweight individuals have a higher risk of developing a post-operative infection, pressure sores, and blood clots in the legs. On the other hand, you should gain weight if you are too thin. Undernourished individuals also have a higher risk of developing a post-operative infection and wound-healing problems. Have your doctor help you stop taking narcotics and muscle relaxants prior to surgery.

The last measure helps you tolerate anesthesia better and gives you better relief from post-operative pain medication. Make sure you cooperate with your primary care physician to obtain all the appropriate pre-operative tests and his or her medical clearance for your surgery. Have all of this information ready for the anesthesiologist, who should also clear you for surgery before you come in the hospital. Overall, the success rate for disc surgery is high and the risk rate is low, so you should not be unnecessarily frightened by the prospect of disc surgery if you have taken the precautions listed above.

One of my patients wrote me the following email, and both she and I thought you would benefit from hearing her story. It illustrates the dilemma that patients and doctors have in deciding when and if to operate for a herniated disc. The story is not uncommon and is quoted directly from her e-mail to me:

> *I have had back problems on and off for the past fifteen years. The only time I was symptom free for a long period of time was when I regularly walked five miles four or five times a week. Starting last March I started having lower back pain, and an MRI indicated a bulging disc. I received physical therapy which helped relieve the pain and then on September 10 when getting out of my car I had such excruciating pain that I had to be treated in the emergency room and did not obtain relief until I received an injection of Toradol, Demerol and Valium. A subsequent MRI revealed a large herniated disc at L-5-S1 level. I was seen by you in early October and received an epidural, which did not relieve the pain. I remember you said WOW when you saw my films. I had a very important interview scheduled for October 19 and I was wondering how I would get through it with all the pain I was having. You suggested taking two Celebrex the night before and it worked. I got through the interview and the pain did not return until that evening. I was in such intense pain that radiated down my right leg that at my request you scheduled surgery for me on October 26. Hurricane Wilma hit on October 24 and I assumed that all elective*

surgery had been canceled. You rescheduled my surgery for the following week. Since my office was closed due to loss of power, the week after the hurricane I stayed at home and got a lot of bed rest. I came down with a terrible cold, which resulted in cancellation of the surgery again because I could not get cleared for anesthesia. By that time my pain was subsiding and I decided to hold off on the surgery. My pain is essentially gone and the only symptom I have now is some numbness in my right foot. You were always persuading me to hold off on the surgery if I could, and I am glad I did. Thank you, Dr. Brown!

This story is typical of the natural course of disc herniations. If you can wait out the symptoms, over 80 percent of the time they will resolve spontaneously. The symptoms resolve because the body has defense mechanisms that dissolve that part of the disc that is herniated out of place.

In the next chapter I will discuss spinal stenosis, a condition that most commonly results from advanced disc degeneration. Like disc herniation, spinal stenosis is a common cause of back and extremity pain. Unlike disc herniation, which is more common in middle-aged people, spinal stenosis occurs more often as we get older. It is a very common cause of back and leg pain in people over the age of 60, yet hardly any of those who suffer from spinal stenosis know what it is!

CHAPTER 6

Spinal Stenosis: What Is It and What Can You Do About It?

What is spinal stenosis? How does it occur? How do I know I have it? If I have it what can I expect? What can I do about it?

Spinal stenosis literally means constriction or narrowing of the spinal canal. Most commonly it is the result of the disc going flat from aging. To understand how disc degeneration leads to spinal stenosis, we need to look at how the spinal canal is built.

Attached to the back of your vertebrae are bony arches. These bony arches are comprised of the walls (pedicles) and the roof (lamina) of your spinal canal. Attached to the bony arch are the bones that project to the sides, called the transverse processes, and those that project to the back, called spinous processes. These

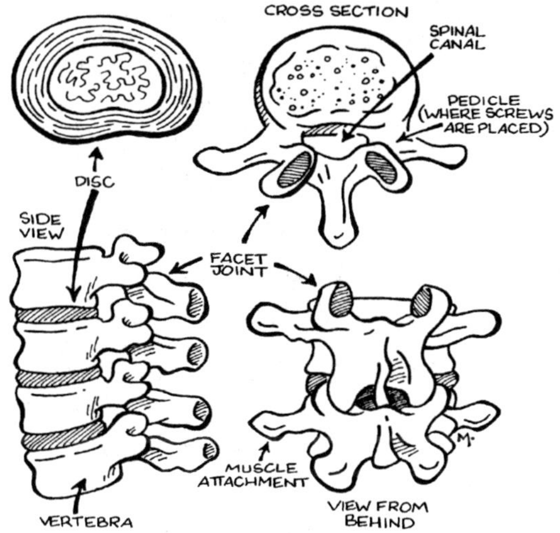

This illustration of the anatomy of the spine from the side, cross section, and from behind shows the relationship of the disc and facet joints to the spinal canal that contains the nerves.

processes are for attachment of the muscles of your spine. Finally there are bones on either side that project upward toward your head and down toward your feet at each vertebra, the facet processes. The facet processes from one vertebra form a joint, about the size of the joint in your thumb, with the facet processes of an adjacent vertebra. These joints are called facet joints, and they are located just behind and to the side of the spinal canal at the level of the disc space. If you look at the cross section of a spine through the disc space, you will see that the spinal canal is surrounded by the disc in front and the facet joints to the back and sides. There are also ligaments, which are strong attachments between bones, like the ACL (anterior cruciate ligament) in your knee, that keep the vertebrae together. They are located just in front of the spinal canal and behind it as well.

How do changes in these structures cause spinal stenosis? (See illustrations on pages 71, 73). As a degenerated disc becomes flat, it bulges and causes the bony arches of the vertebrae to come together. This in turn causes the facet joints to be pushed out of alignment and then become arthritic and enlarged. As the disc narrows, the ligaments of the spine become shortened and thick. All of these consequences of the disc degeneration, along with the bulge of the disc itself, result in narrowing of the spinal canal and nerve channels that contain the nerves going to your arms and legs.

How constricted does the spinal canal become? The size of the normal spinal canal in your low back can be pictured by making a circle with your thumb and index finger the diameter of a quarter. Now decrease the size of the circle to the diameter of a pencil to illustrate severe spinal stenosis. Picture all of the nerves for the muscles and the sensation in your legs as well as for your bowel, bladder, and sexual function going through the normal quarter-sized-diameter spinal canal, with some room to spare. Then picture these nerves being squeezed into a spinal canal the diameter of a pencil, with no room at all to spare. That is severe spinal stenosis. A combination of bulging of the disc, thickening of the spinal ligaments, and arthritic enlargement of the facet joints and vertebrae (osteophytes, or "bone spurs") can constrict the spinal canal to the diameter of a pencil, thus preventing oxygen from reaching the spinal nerves.

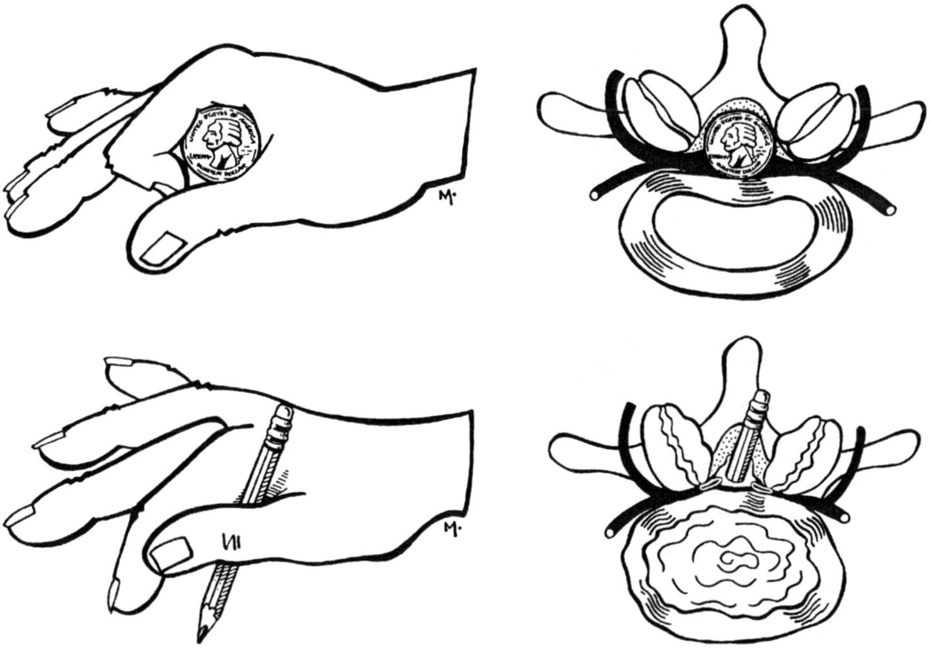

The normal diameter of the spinal canal on the low back is the size of a quarter, whereas the severely constricted spinal canal from spinal stenosis is the diameter of a pencil.

How does spinal stenosis cause pain?

Your spinal nerves can withstand a lot of compression if it is applied slowly and evenly. Therefore they can be squeezed pretty tightly before they become painful. However, as you walk the nerves normally glide back and forth in your spinal canal. This gliding action is restricted as the spinal canal becomes tighter. Because the spinal nerves cannot glide normally, they become irritated and swell up, taking up even more room in an already tight spinal canal. This, in turn, causes the nerves to produce pain impulses that are perceived by the brain to be from your legs.

How do I know I have spinal stenosis?

You should suspect spinal stenosis in your low back if you have aching pain in your legs brought on by walking and relieved by sitting (neurogenic claudication). The pain may be localized to your back, or it may radiate from your back to one or both legs, buttocks, thighs, even as far as your calves and your feet. The symptoms of spinal stenosis in your back may be pain in any combination of the locations mentioned above,

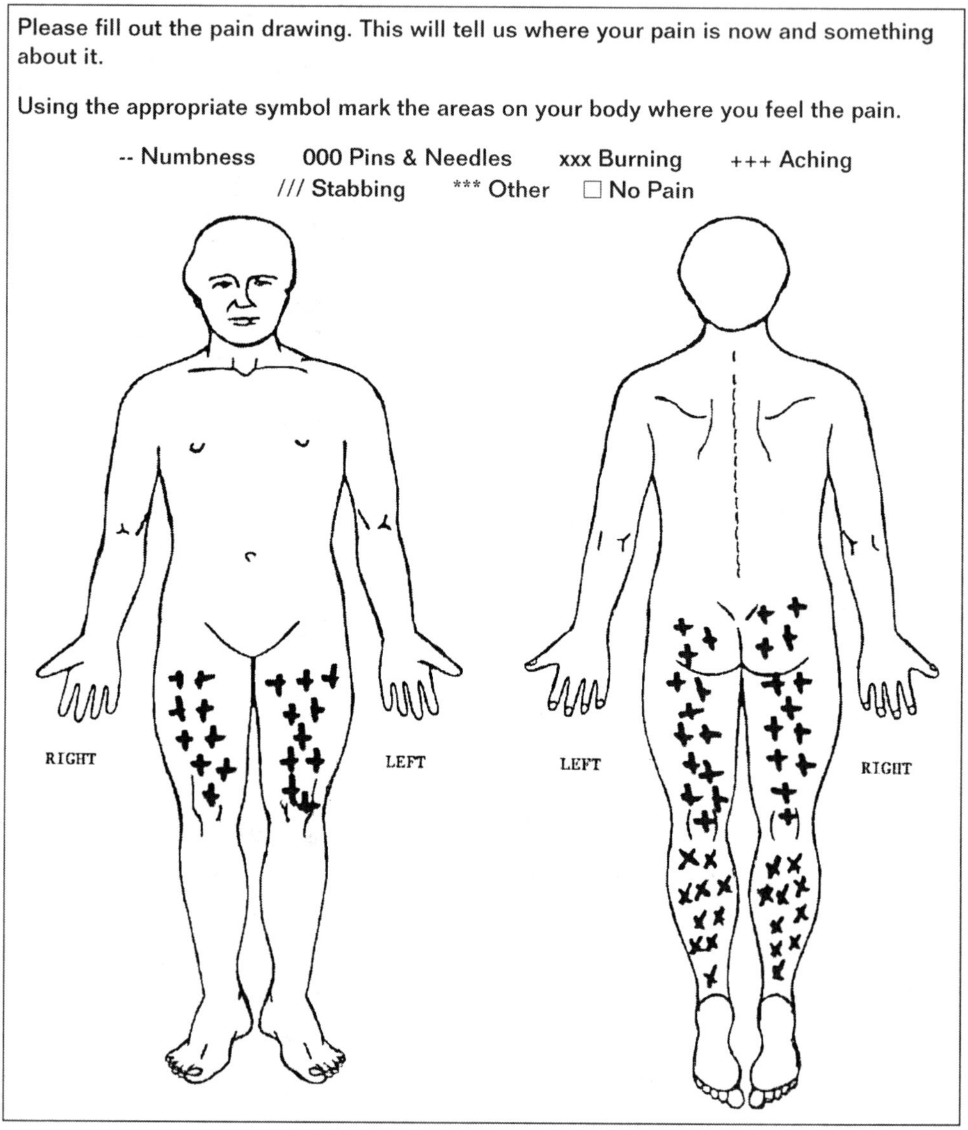

This patient-generated pain drawing depicts pain from spinal stenosis in the back of the legs and front of the thighs (symbol for aching is + sign) and pain from poor circulation in the calves (symbol for burning is the X sign).

depending on the level(s), degrees of constriction, and sites of the spinal stenosis. At each of the five discs in your low back there are five sites at which constriction can take place. Spinal stenosis in the central spinal canal causes classic aching pain in the front and back of your thighs and calves.

At each disc level in your spine, the nerve channels can be constricted at two locations on each side, as well as in the spinal canal itself. On either side of your spinal canal the nerves can be squeezed where they begin to exit the spinal canal (lateral recess stenosis, see illustration on page 71), in the channel through which the nerve exits the spinal canal (foraminal stenosis). Therefore there are 25 possible sites at which the nerves to your legs can be entrapped by spinal stenosis, in your low back alone!

More often than not, by the time you develop symptoms from spinal stenosis, the nerves are being squeezed at more than one site at the same time. I will explain how we determine exactly where the pain is coming from later in this chapter.

The classic symptoms of spinal stenosis – aching in the legs with walking that is relieved by rest (neurogenic claudication) – can be confused with the symptoms caused by poor circulation in your legs (vascular claudication). If you have poor blood circulation in your legs, walking may cause aching in your legs that is relieved by rest, very similar to the symptoms seen with spinal stenosis, but with some important differences. When the muscles in your legs do not get enough oxygen because of poor circulation, they produce lactic acid with activity. Lactic acid produces cramping pain in the muscles (see figure page 74).

How do I know my pain is from spinal stenosis and not from poor circulation?

There are some subtle differences in symptoms between the pain from spinal stenosis and poor circulation. Pain from spinal stenosis usually begins in the low back and radiates into the leg(s) and is relieved by sitting or bending over; both maneuvers open up the spinal canal, thus relieving the pressure on the nerves. Patients are frequently confused by the symptoms of spinal stenosis because their walking is limited by leg pain but they are still able to bicycle, dance, or lean on a shopping cart and get around without pain. All of these postures allow the person to bend forward enough to open up the spinal canal, relieving the pressure on their spinal nerves. When you see someone who is having difficulty walking because of spinal stenosis, they usually walk in a characteristic bent-forward position. Patients with spinal stenosis will tell you that they have good days when they can walk unlimited distances and bad days when their walking is very limited.

The symptoms of poor circulation to the legs start as a cramping sensation in the calves and radiate proximally upward into the whole leg. The pain is not relieved by bending forward. The symptoms progress with physical activity as the lactic acid in the oxygen-starved muscles builds up. The person experiencing these symptoms would rather stand than sit for relief because blood flow to the legs is stronger while standing than sitting. They cannot walk, bicycle, dance, or take part in any physical activity without developing muscle pain. The symptoms of vascular claudication are the same every day.

Spinal stenosis and poor circulation to the legs are more common after the age of 60 and can occur simultaneously, so it is possible to have symptoms of both conditions at the same time. I have seen patients who could clearly describe to me the symptoms of both. I can advise these folks which symptom is coming from which condition, and then determine from them which pain they more urgently want to be relieved of. Most people can tolerate vascular claudication better than neurogenic claudication and want their spinal stenosis fixed first. However, your PCP should refer you to a vascular surgeon to help you decide whether to pursue surgery for vascular claudicaton.

How is the pain from spinal stenosis different from a herniated disc?

Sciatic leg pain from a herniated disc can sometimes be confused with pain from spinal stenosis. It is important to distinguish which condition the symptoms stem from because herniated discs will usually shrink with time and the pain will resolve on its own, whereas the symptoms from spinal stenosis may gradually become worse over time and eventually require surgery for relief. Disc herniations, as you will recall from Chapter 5, produce pain by compressing, stretching, and chemically irritating the spinal nerve. Leg pain from a herniated disc usually radiates along the course of a spinal nerve and is present even at rest. In contrast, the pain from spinal stenosis radiates over the course of more than one nerve and is relieved by sitting or bending over. The ability to bend over at the waist while standing and to lift the symptomatic leg up while lying face up is limited by a herniated disc. Bending and straight-leg raising are not limited and in fact may relieve the pain from spinal stenosis.

A disc herniation may contribute to spinal stenosis, particularly when it occurs in the lateral recess or foramen of the spinal canal. This can happen when a disc herniation occurs in a small or misshapen spinal canal. The normal spinal canal is triangular in shape and the diameter of a quarter. Approximately 10 percent of people are born with a cloverleaf-shaped spinal canal that approaches the size of a nickel or smaller. This is called congenital spinal stenosis. Smaller degenerative changes in the disc and facet joints may result in more significant encroachment on a misshapen or small spinal canal than they would on a normally shaped and sized spinal canal. This is particularly true in the lateral recess, that area on the side of the spinal canal where the nerves just begin to enter the channel to exit the canal. A small disc bulge or herniation in a congenitally small lateral recess may result in severe leg pain, whereas it would cause no symptoms in a normal lateral recess. Lateral-recess stenosis with a disc herniation may cause a combination of the classic symptoms and physical findings seen with either condition alone.

A typical symptom of lateral-recess stenosis is leg pain with rotation of the spine, such as at the end of a golf swing. I once operated on a famous professional golfer who had pain at the end of her golf swing that was seriously affecting her ability to compete. I performed a surgical decompression of one lateral recess and she was able to continue playing on the international circuit. I took care of a college soccer player who had sciatic leg pain when he kicked the ball. He had spinal stenosis localized to one lateral recess. I surgically decompressed his lateral recess and he went on to become a professional player in Europe.

Other causes of spinal stenosis

Constriction of the spinal canal can result from conditions other than disc degeneration, congenital small canal, and disc herniation. Cysts can form on degenerated facet joints similar to the cysts that form on arthritic finger joints. They are called facet-joint cysts or synovial cysts of the facet joint. These cysts can cause spinal stenosis and produce aching symptoms in the legs. They usually occur in the lumbar spine, but I have seen them in the cervical and thoracic spine as well. They are benign, not cancerous, and rarely recur after they are surgically removed.

Paget's disease is a condition that causes bones to thicken and joints to become arthritic. Paget's disease can involve the vertebrae, facet joints, and lamina of the spine, resulting in a severe form of spinal stenosis.

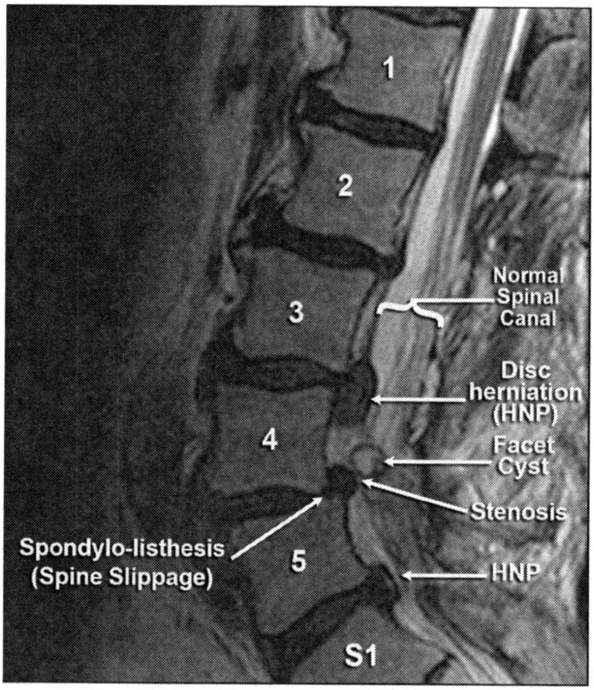

This MRI scan of the low back, side view, shows the spinal canal that has been constricted (spinal stenosis) by a bulging disc, slippage of the spine, and a facet joint cyst. There are two other herniated discs (HNP), one large and one smaller. It is unusual to see all of these conditions in the same patient.

Very slow-growing benign tumors of the nerves inside the spinal canal (neurofibroma, schwannoma) can constrict the space for the remaining nerves and cause symptoms typical of spinal stenosis. However, these tumors are usually associated with progressively severe night pain that disturbs normal sleep patterns. Although most people have night pain with spinal stenosis, it is relieved by certain positions, such as sleeping on your side with your legs curled up.

Some small people, such as those born with achondroplasia, can have an extremely small spinal canal and develop the symptoms of spinal stenosis as early as in their teens.

Not even the doctors agree if the pain is from my back or my hip

The symptoms of spinal stenosis in the upper lumbar spine between the first, second, and third lumbar discs can be confused with symptoms coming from an arthritic hip or knee joint. Since spinal stenosis most commonly occurs in the age groups who suffer from arthritis of these joints, symptoms can be coming from the spine and joint arthritis at the same time. I published a study of the symptoms of 97 patients who had symptoms of spinal stenosis alone, symptoms of hip arthritis alone, or symptoms of spinal stenosis and hip arthritis together. The study showed that if you have groin pain and a limp with loss of motion in the hip, you are more apt to have hip arthritis. If you have a positive femoral-stretch test, which means you have pain in the front of your thigh when you bend your knee while lying on your stomach, you are more likely to have spinal stenosis. A combination of these findings would suggest that both conditions are symptomatic at the same time.

A patient once consulted me because of back pain, aching in her legs while walking, a limp, groin pain, and loss of motion in one hip. She had an MRI scan of her spine that showed spinal stenosis and an x-ray of her hip that showed osteoarthritis. She was exercising for an hour a day on an exercise bicycle and had lost 50 pounds on a diet over the previous year. Her quality of life was moderately impaired because she could no longer play tennis. She did not want to have her hip replaced or have spinal surgery for stenosis. Her reason for the consultation was to get my reassurance that she was not harming herself by delaying surgery on her spine. I reassured her that, on the contrary, she was helping herself by exercising and waiting for surgery until either condition significantly impaired her quality of life. If she had been unable to keep up her exercise routine and was getting out of shape, I would have recommended surgery for her hip as well as her spine. The order in which I would

Please fill out the pain drawing. This will tell us where your pain is now and something about it.

Using the appropriate symbol mark the areas on your body where you feel the pain.

-- Numbness   000 Pins & Needles   xxx Burning   +++ Aching
/// Stabbing   *** Other   ☐ No Pain

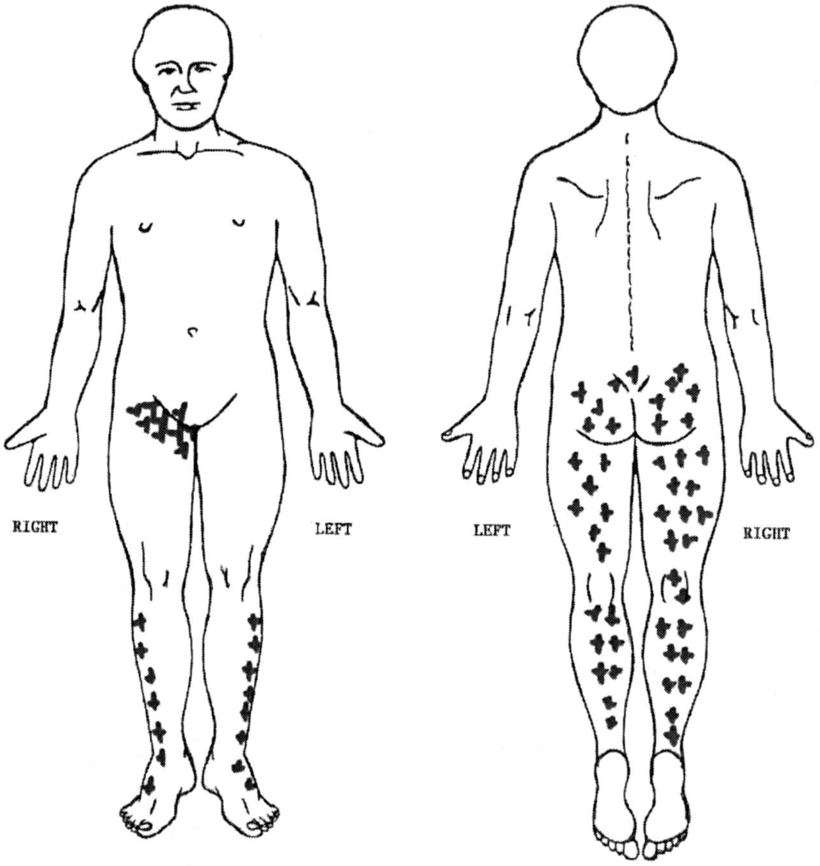

In this pain drawing, the patient shows pain in the right groin from arthritis of the right hip and pain down the backs of the legs and sides of the thighs from spinal stenosis in the low back. The patient describes the pain from both conditions as aching in nature.

have recommended the surgery, hip versus spine, would have depended on which symptoms were bothering her most – those coming from the hip or those coming from the spine.

Symptoms of spinal stenosis in the low back, neck, and both places at the same time

Twenty percent of people with symptomatic spinal stenosis in the lumbar spine (low back) can have stenosis in the cervical spine (neck). The normal diameter of the spinal canal in the neck is the size of a nickel. The spinal cord in the neck is the diameter of a dime. The combination of disc narrowing and bulging, facet enlargement, and ligament thickening can narrow the spinal canal in the neck to less than the diameter of the spinal cord. When this occurs, the blood supply to the spinal cord in the neck can be shut off and parts of the spinal cord will stop functioning (myelopathy). This is exactly what happened to my aunt (read her story in Chapter 1).

Loss of balance, stumbling, tripping, falling, and lack of coordination may be symptoms of spinal stenosis in the neck. Although some patients will experience pain in the arms with exercise that is relieved by rest (neurogenic claudication), it is not as common as leg pain from spinal stenosis in the low back. This presents a real problem for patients who have severe symptomatic spinal stenosis in the neck and low back at the same time. Occasionally I will see a patient with severe spinal stenosis in the low back and neck who cannot walk more than a few hundred feet because of leg pain. They are so preoccupied with their leg pain that they do not realize that they are tripping and falling because of severe spinal stenosis in their neck. I try to explain to them that they should have an operation on their neck to relieve the pressure on their spinal cord to prevent paralysis (remember the story of my aunt whose surgery was too late to save her?) before having an operation on their low back to relieve their leg pain. This is always difficult for the individual to understand because they want their pain relieved first. Fortunately, for some people who are in good general health, we can perform surgery on the neck and the low back under the same anesthesia.

Spinal stenosis in the neck, rotator cuff pain, and carpal tunnel syndrome

Arm pain from a spinal stenosis or a disc herniation in the neck can be confused with shoulder pain from rotator-cuff problems and with hand pain from carpal tunnel syndrome. All three conditions may be present at the same time, with pain from one site compounding the pain from another site and confusing the patient as well as the doctor as to where the pain is coming from. This situation is called shoulder-hand syndrome. In these cases I will consult a neurologist (medical specialist in diseases of the brain, spinal cord, and peripheral nerves; see Chapter 4) to try to determine which site is the primary source of the arm pain. Neurologists often perform an electomyogram and nerve conduction velocity (EMG/NCV) to sort out this syndrome. This test is performed by placing needles in your muscles and stimulating the nerves to the muscles and measuring the way the muscle contracts as well as the speed of the impulse along the stimulated nerve. An EMG/NCV can determine if the pain is coming from the nerve being stimulated in the neck area or at the wrist (carpel tunnel syndrome). It is an uncomfortable test, but it is not harmful or dangerous. This test is also used to differentiate leg pain from peripheral neuropathy, a condition seen in diabetics, versus pain from spinal stenosis.

Another source of pain in the upper extremities that can be confused with spinal stenosis is thoracic outlet syndrome, which is a constriction of nerves from your neck to your arm that occurs between your collarbone and your first rib at the base of your neck. This is a rare syndrome and can be diagnosed by your doctor by feeling the arterial pulses in your wrists at the same time your arm is moved passively throughout a range of motion.

Spinal stenosis can also occur in the thoracic spine, but it is rare. If it does occur, it is usually localized to the lower thoracic spine where it joins the lumbar spine. And it is almost always associated with spinal stenosis in the lumbar spine. The symptoms of spinal stenosis in the thoracic spine can be pain and weakness in the legs with walking. Anyone with a congenitally small spinal canal is susceptible to developing symptomatic spinal stenosis in the thoracic spine. Therefore we usually perform an MRI scan of the entire spine, neck, chest, and low back in people who are born with a small spinal canal.

When should I have surgery for spinal stenosis?

Is surgery the only answer for spinal stenosis? Let's answer that question for the low back first. Spinal stenosis develops slowly over a period of years and usually does not cause nerve damage. Symptoms of pain, weakness, or poor balance may come on intermittently and slowly or all at once near the end stage of the disease, when the spinal canal is severely narrowed. From my experience in advising thousands of patients who suffer from the symptoms of spinal stenosis, surgery is appropriate when the quality of life of the individual has significantly deteriorated. Most patients do not want to undergo surgery until their walking is impaired to the point that they cannot walk more than two city blocks. This degree of impairment usually corresponds to a significant deterioration in the person's quality of life. Patients who cannot sit comfortably, walk short distances, stand for any period of time, and whose sleep is impaired because of pain usually request surgery, and that is when it is indicated.

What is the surgery, how is it performed, and what results can I expect from it?

Spinal stenosis is corrected surgically by performing laminectomies and foraminotomies at each constricted level. This means that the roof of the spinal canal (lamina) and part of the enlarged facet joints are removed along with the thickened ligaments to decompress the spinal canal and nerve channels (foramen). To adequately decompress the constricted spinal canal requires open surgery in my experience. I have had to re-operate on many patients who previously had micro- or arthroscopic surgery for spinal stenosis. The corrective surgery following these minimal procedures is much more difficult and the results are not as good as they could have been had the person had effective surgery from the beginning.

The necessity for emergency surgery for spinal stenosis is rare in my experience. Over the past 35 years of taking care of patients with this condition, I have had to perform emergency surgery on very few patients with spinal stenosis. One patient fell in the bathtub and ruptured a disc in a very constricted spinal canal, causing cauda equina syndrome. Another patient with severe spinal stenosis had an acute onset of paralysis following an epidural steroid injection. I do not prescribe epidurals for patients with severe spinal stenosis for this reason. And I have also performed surgery on several patients with spinal stenosis that was made acutely worse as the

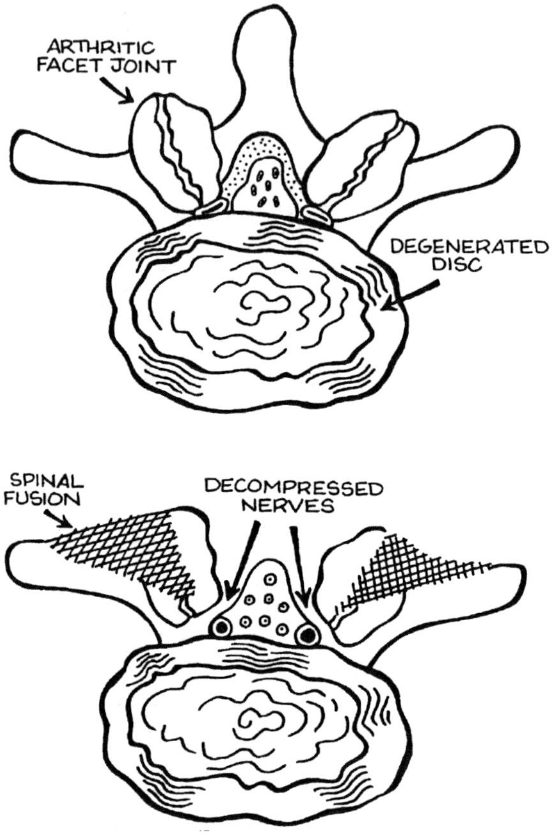

Top drawing shows spinal stenosis with pinched nerve. Bottom drawing shows the nerves decompressed, and the crosshatches show the location of a spinal fusion.

result of a vertebral fracture where bone was displaced into an already constricted spinal canal.

As I stated in the previous chapter, the size of a disc herniation on the MRI scan should not be an indication for surgical disc excision. On the contrary, the appearance of spinal stenosis on an MRI is one indication for surgery for this disorder. Research shows that when there is more than 75 percent constriction of the spinal canal in a person whose activity is limited by pain, surgery is the best way to obtain relief. This is particularly true when the spinal canal is highly constricted at more than one disc level, which is usually the situation. Spinal stenosis usually is most common between the fourth and fifth and the third and fourth vertebrae on the low back, and between the fifth and sixth and the sixth and seventh vertebrae in the neck. It is common for spinal stenosis to occur at more than one disc level in both the neck and low back.

Does all spinal stenosis require surgery for relief?

I have managed many more patients with symptomatic spinal stenosis without surgery than I have operated upon. The best long-term treatment is any aerobic exercise that you can perform for at least 30 minutes daily within the limits of your pain and stamina. Walking, either outside or on a treadmill, riding a stationary bicycle, and aquatic exercises are the best aerobic exercises. You should do whichever one you can tolerate the best. I do not recommend stretching, massage, traction, or manipulation for patients with spinal stenosis. These maneuvers can aggravate the pain coming from the low back and increase the pressure on the spinal cord in the neck.

Maintaining a nutritious and healthy diet is as important for your back as it is for your blood pressure, brain, and heart. If you are overweight, you should lose weight to take the pressure off of your back. And if you are underweight, try to eat the correct foods to maintain your bone strength. Much more will be said about these issues in Chapter 11. Eating nutritiously and maintaining a healthy weight will help you to live with spinal stenosis and avoid surgery. Even if you eventually require surgery for this condition, maintaining normal weight, strength, and stamina will increase your chances of excellent results.

Spinal stenosis may be aggravated or caused by deformities of the spine such as curvature (scoliosis) or slippage of the spine (spondylolisthesis) – more about these conditions in the next chapter.

CHAPTER 7

What To Do If Your Pain Is From an Unstable or Deformed Spine

One in 20 people in North America have the inherited form of spondylolisthesis (slippage of the spine).

The most common deformity of the spine that can cause back pain or contribute to the severity of painful spinal stenosis is spondylolisthesis. You have

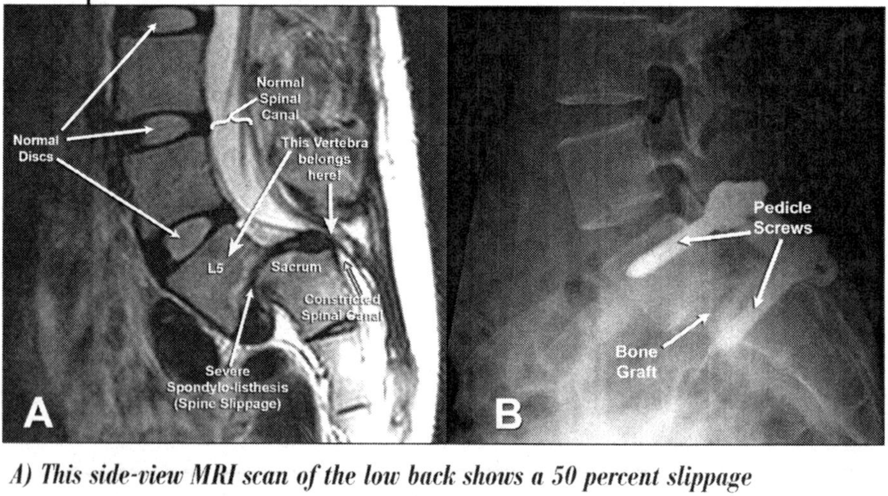

A) This side-view MRI scan of the low back shows a 50 percent slippage (spondylolisthesis) of the L5 vertebra on the sacrum. The spinal canal is highly constricted from the slippage, which caused this patient to have a lot of leg pain and difficulty walking. B) Side-view x-ray of the same patient's low back, one year after a bone graft was used to correct the slippage. The bone graft was held in place with pedicle screws and rods.

conquered half of this book when you can say spondy-lo-lis-thesis rapidly! Spondylolisthesis literally means spine (spondy) and slippage (listhesis). Literally, one vertebra slips forward on the one below. Just as with spinal stenosis, there are two forms of spondylolisthesis: the first one, isthmic spondylolisthesis, is inherited; and the other is secondary to disc degeneration, degenerative spondylolisthesis (occurs as a result of disc degeneration, see illustration on page 78).

One in 20 people in North America have the inherited form of spondylolisthesis. It most commonly occurs between the fifth lumbar vertebra and the sacrum (L5-S1) in your low back, coincidentally the most common level for disc herniation (see Chapter 5). It rarely occurs at other levels of the lumbar spine and in the neck. The inherited defect that allows the fifth vertebra to slip forward on the sacrum is in the bony arch that I described to you in Chapter 6. The defect occurs in the part that connects the superior articular process to the inferior articular process (pars interarticularis defect, a.k.a. pars defect). This defect, with or without a slippage of the vertebra, first appears in the second decade of life between the ages of 10 and 20 years. It is usually discovered on x-ray when a young person complains of back pain. However, most of the time it is painless and a person does not know they have it.

One of my colleague's sons was a college football player who was complaining of back pain. I examined him and thought I could feel a step off between the two lowest spinous processes in his low back. An x-ray of his spine confirmed my suspicion that he had spondylolisthesis at L5-S1. I let him continue playing football while wearing a corset, and his back pain eventually went away on its own. He is now in his 40s and rarely complains about his back.

There are all degrees of spondylolisthesis, from just a defect in the pars to total slippage of the fifth vertebra off of the sacrum and into the pelvis (spondyloloptosis – you do not even have to try and say this word), a very difficult condition to treat for the patient as well as the doctor. I have only had to treat two patients with this condition in my career. Most patients have between a 25 and 50 percent slippage. The degree of slippage does not determine whether the condition is painful. Back pain may develop if the slippage makes the spine susceptible to repeated sprains. The most common reason why spondylolisthesis becomes painful is secondary to spinal stenosis, which usually occurs after the age of 40 when the disc at the slipped level degenerates and narrows.

Degenerative spondylolisthesis (acquired) is when the slippage occurs because of disc narrowing as the result of degeneration. There are no inherited bony defects to cause this type of slippage. Degenerative spondylolisthesis occurs most commonly in women over the age of 60 at the L4-5 level of the lumbar spine. It can also occur in the other disc levels of the lumbar spine; in fact, it can occur at several levels at the same time. In the neck it is most commonly seen at the C4-5 level. I have seen only one case of it in the thoracic spine.

Degenerative spondylolisthesis is more commonly associated with spinal stenosis than is inherited spondylolisthesis. To visualize how either type of slippage of the spine contributes to spinal stenosis, superimpose a circle made by apposing your thumb and index finger the size of a quarter on your right hand over the same-sized circle on your left hand. Now slide your right hand over your left hand and notice how the passageway through the circles decreases in size. The same thing happens in the spinal canal, which becomes constricted (stenotic) when one vertebra slips forward on the adjacent one. Superimpose a bulging degenerated disc over a spinal canal that has already been constricted from slippage of adjacent vertebrae and you can see how the two conditions compound one another to make the stenosis worse.

Back and leg pain occurs from degenerative spondylolisthesis because of susceptibility of the spine to repeated sprains and secondarily to constriction of the nerve channels The back pain is mechanical in nature, meaning it is brought on by lifting and bending and is relieved by rest. The leg pain is typical neurogenic claudication seen with spinal stenosis (see Chapter 6).

The presence of either type of slippage of the spine implies that the spine is inherently unstable, which makes it susceptible to painful sprains and to worsening of the slippage. Therefore slippage of the spine is the most common reason for a surgical spinal fusion (scan B on page 86), the process of solidly fixing one vertebra to another with metal devices and a bone graft (more about spinal fusion on page 93). A fusion is performed for spondylolisthesis to relieve chronic mechanical low-back pain as well as to prevent the slippage from getting worse. When surgery is required to relieve pain from spinal stenosis, a fusion is almost always recommended and necessary for satisfactory long-term relief of back pain (see illustration, page 84).

What does it mean that my spine is unstable?

Instability of the spine, a.k.a. unstable spine or mechanical insufficiency of the spine, means that the spine is unable to function under normal stresses and maintain normal alignment and/or protect the nerves within. Spinal instability can cause neurogenic, arthritic, mechanical, and fatigue pain. The unstable spine is susceptible to repeated sprains and strains, just as someone with an unstable ankle is susceptible to repeated ankle sprains. The unstable spine is also susceptible to slipping or curving more. Instability of the spine can be caused by inherited defects such as spondylolisthesis, disc degeneration, and destructive lesions of bone such as fractures, tumors, and infections.

The diagnosis of spinal instability is made with bending x-rays (stress x-rays), which include a standing side-view x-ray (lateral) while you stand straight, while you bend forward (flexion), and then while you bend backward (extension). The displacement between your vertebrae in these three postures is compared in order to determine change in angulations and slippages. When one vertebra's position changes more than is normal compared to the adjacent vertebra, then that segment of the spine is considered unstable. You can imagine that the nerves can easily be pinched by abnormal movement if a constricted spine is too loose. Instability of the spine causes spinal stenosis to be more painful. People who suffer from this combination in their low back will frequently complain of pain shifting from one leg to the other and back again for no apparent reason. The reason is that with rotation of the spine the nerve is pinched first on one side then the other.

Scoliosis (curvature of the spine)

Like spondylolisthesis, scoliosis — or curvature of the spine — comes in two major varieties: inherited and acquired (degenerative). Curvature

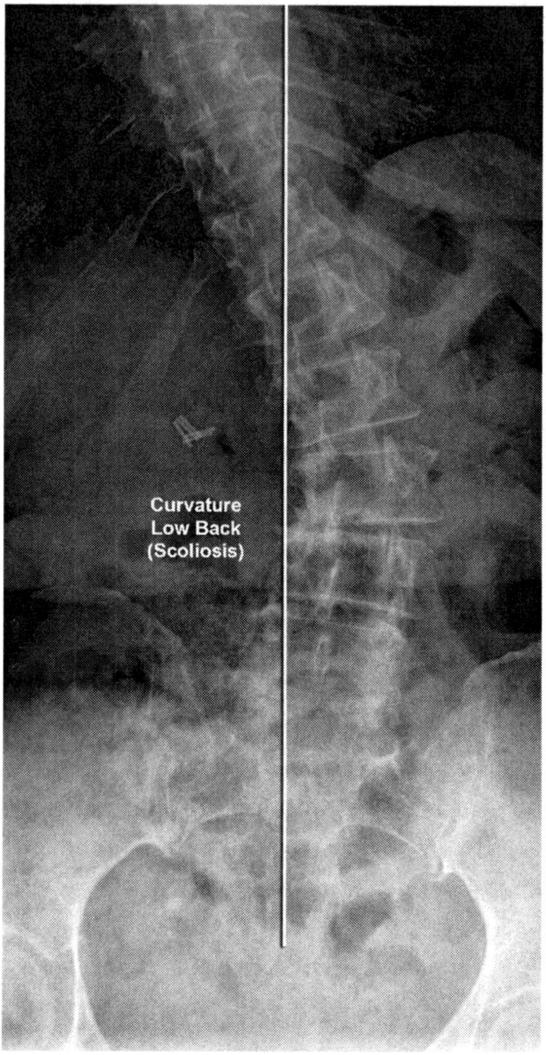

This front-view low-back x-ray shows curvature of the spine; note how the disc is now on the concave side of the curve.

of the spine can also cause muscular fatigue as well as neurogenic pain. When your body is thrown off of balance by a curvature (your head is not directly located over your pelvis), your muscles continually work to straighten up your back. They become fatigued and painful in the process. When scoliosis produces pain in adolescents it is usually the result of muscle fatigue, whereas pain from spinal curvature in adults is usually the result of nerve pressure from spinal stenosis, mechanical pain (instability of the spine and susceptibility to sprains), and muscle fatigue. Spinal fusion with metal fixation devices is performed for painful scoliosis to correct the deformity and to maintain that correction, as well as to prevent future worsening of the curvature.

Some older adults have a combination of constriction (spinal stenosis), slippage (spondylolisthesis), curvature (scoliosis), and instability of the spine at the same time! These four conditions can also produce nerve, mechanical, and muscle fatigue pain at the same time. When all three conditions are present, it is almost always necessary to perform a surgical decompression of the constricted spinal canal and spinal fusion with metal screws and rods, as well as bone grafting in order to obtain long-lasting relief of pain. The combination of these painful disorders of the spine and the necessity for a major (certainly not micro!) operation to obtain relief is difficult to explain to a person in their 80s. I have seen patients who have tried to get by with smaller, less-invasive "micro" operations for these conditions, but they received little pain relief from the procedure and were after that almost impossible to help. If your doctor tells you that your pain is coming from any one or any combination of these conditions and that you can be treated with micro-surgery, I advise you to obtain a second opinion from a qualified spinal surgeon (see Chapter 4).

Inherited curvature of the spine comes in several varieties. The most common curvature under the age of 18 is idiopathic adolescent scoliosis (curvature of the spine in adolescence, the cause of which is unknown). The term idiopathic is old terminology when it comes to adolescent scoliosis because we now know that this type of curvature is inherited. These curves are not present at birth but begin to form at the beginning of the growth spurt, age nine to 14 in girls and 11 to 15 in boys. They are usually detected in school scoliosis screening programs. If you get notice from the school that your growing daughter or son has scoliosis, do not panic; the majority of these cases require no treatment. However, you should have your pediatrician follow the progress of the curve to determine if it needs to be treated. Your pediatrician will refer you to a children's scoliosis specialist (pediatric orthopaedic spine specialist) if it is necessary for the scoliosis to be followed or treated with a brace or surgery.

Two myths that must be dispelled are that exercise will correct or keep a curvature of the spine from getting worse, and that the curvature occurs because of bad posture. The truth is that curvature of the spine and the degree to which an adolescent curvature advances are determined by genetic factors (similar to adolescent disc degeneration – see Chapter 1). Therefore, all the good posture and exercise in the world will not prevent or correct curvature of the spine in adolescents. Blaming the curvature on poor posture or insisting that your daughter or son exercise to correct a scoliosis is futile and wrong. The presence and progression of the curvature is genetically programmed. A better approach is to explain to your young person that maintaining good health will help them obtain a better result from treatment of their scoliosis, be it a brace or surgery.

The other two types of inherited scoliosis are congenital scoliosis (an inherited type of curvature of the spine that is present from birth and detected before the age of two) and infantile scoliosis (occurs between two and nine years of age). These forms of scoliosis should be managed by a pediatric orthopaedic specialist in a children's hospital setting. Most of these curves require sophisticated surgical correction at an early age, and there should be no delay in finding appropriate care for the child or infant with scoliosis.

Infants and young children do not complain of pain from scoliosis. Adolescents complain of aching and fatigue when the curvature reaches a certain severity and/or causes them to be out of balance. When a young person of any age complains of spine pain, particularly if it causes sleep disturbance, it could indicate a more serious problem and they should be seen by their pediatrician for evaluation as soon as possible. If a young person is sick and has a fever or a stiff neck along with neck, chest, or back pain, they should be taken for emergency care immediately.

There is a certain peculiar painful condition of the spine that occurs in adolescents and can cause muscle spasm and scoliosis. This condition, called osteoid osteoma, is a small bone reaction about the size of a pea that can be located anywhere in the spine and causes severe night pain, which is dramatically relieved by aspirin. It is not a tumor, but it is so painful that it causes the spine to lean over like the Leaning Tower of Pisa. The diagnosis is made by finding a dense circle of bone on an x-ray near where the patient complains of pain. A test called a bone scan shows a very dark spot over the skeleton. I once took care of a 14-year-old young man with this condition who was dramatically cured of his pain and curvature by removing the pea-sized lesion with a large biopsy needle using fluoroscopy, a moving x-ray imaging system. He no longer had to take aspirin to be able to sleep, and his spinal curvature went away.

Osteoporosis and back pain

A common cause of deformity and spine pain is osteoporosis, or softening of the bones. Osteoporosis is most commonly seen in small, post-menopausal women, particularly those who have a history of smoking. When the bone becomes soft, the vertebrae can collapse from minor trauma, such as riding over a speed bump, and cause kyphosis (excessive rounding of the spine).

If you look at the spine from the side, there are normal curves that balance each other so that the head is centered over the pelvis. In the neck and low back the curve is forward (lordosis), and in the thoracic spine and sacrum (that part that attaches to your pelvis) the spine curves backward (kyphosis). With osteoporotic compression fractures of the vertebrae the spine becomes more rounded, with accentuated kyphosis in the thoracic spine, usually seen in older osteoporotic women. When this occurs in the lumbar spine there is a loss of the normal swayback appearance (loss of lordosis), called flat back. Incidentally, a flat back can also occur as the result of degenerative disc narrowing. Rounding of the spine, be it in the thoracic or lumbar spine, throws the body off balance (tilting it forward) and results in pain from muscle fatigue.

As we humans live longer and more sedentary lives, we become susceptible to all of these conditions. I am seeing more and more patients in their 80s and 90s who have a combination of degenerative narrowed discs, spondylolisthesis, scoliosis, spinal stenosis, and osteoporosis with kyphosis from vertebral fractures. They become totally disabled and some even become wheelchair bound because of neurogenic, arthritic, muscular, and mechanical pain. We can help some of these folks with modern spinal surgery, but it is much better to try to prevent these things from happening in the first place. We must teach our youth to exercise, take enough calcium, and never smoke! More will be said about measures to treat and prevent these painful conditions of the spine in Chapter 11.

What is a spinal fusion, and how will it relieve my pain?

Surgery for spondylolisthesis, scoliosis, kyphosis, and any combination of these spinal deformities is indicated when they cause chronic pain and disability. Deformities cause mechanical pain from instability, nerve pain from spinal stenosis, muscle fatigue pain from spinal imbalance, and arthritic pain from wear and tear on the small joints of the spine as well as the discs.

Spinal fusion is performed by grafting bone from one vertebra to an adjacent vertebra and allowing the bone to heal between these structures. Spinal fusion relieves mechanical pain by taking away the abnormal motion between the vertebrae. It relieves the muscle fatigue pain by maintaining correction of spinal balance, so that you are not leaning over all the time. And it corrects the arthritic pain by taking away the motion in the arthritic joints of the affected spine. Correcting the deformity and fusing the spine can also relieve nerve pain if, in the process, the spinal canal is opened up to some degree.

How are screws, rods, and hooks used in a spinal fusion?

Today we have highly perfected metal implants that are effective in correcting the deformed spine and fixing it tightly until the bone heals and takes over from the metal. The implants are comprised fixation systems made up of any combination of screws, rods, hooks, wires, and plates, which can be made of stainless steel or titanium. These systems are designed for fixation of the spine at any level from your head to your pelvis, from in front, back, or side. They have revolutionized our ability to help people with terribly unstable and deformed spines regain a near-normal quality of life. Modern spinal fixation devices, along with MRI scans and modern anesthesia (more about this later), are the three things that have revolutionized the surgical treatment of most painful spinal disorders.

I should tell you more about the unfairly and infamously labeled pedicle screws because they have revolutionized our ability to safely stabilize the spine. These screws are placed in the pedicles or walls of the spinal canal to be able to attach one vertebra to another vertebra (see x-ray on page 86). Pedicle screws were made infamous in television ads aired all over the United States in the 1990s by lawyers who were soliciting cases for a class-action suit on behalf of patients who had received the screws in their spinal fusions. Allegedly the screws were placed in these patients without a United States Food and Drug Administration (U.S. FDA) new-device approval. Even though the case was eventually thrown out of court, the bad publicity surrounding the spinal screws had already unjustly scared patients concerning them. This is unfortunate, because sometimes the use of pedicle screws is the only reasonable way of fixing a painful spine deformity (see Figure B, page 86). I would personally choose to have pedicle screws placed in my back if I suffered from a problem in which they were indicated. I think they are a safe, effective, and sometimes the only way to treat some painful spinal deformities.

Where do you get the bone for a spinal fusion?

The standard source of the bone graft is from your pelvic bone, the iliac crest (more about bone grafts and bone graft substitutes in a moment). The bone graft is taken from one side of the back of the pelvis for spinal fusions performed from behind the spine and from the front of the pelvis for spinal fusions performed in front of the spine. A second incision may be required to take the bone graft. Many patients complain more about pain at the site the bone graft was taken from than at the site of the spinal fusion.

In patients who require long spinal fusions, particularly those with scoliosis, and in older patients with poor bone quality, it is sometimes impossible to obtain enough of the patient's own bone to perform the fusion. For these and other reasons, bone graft substitutes have been perfected. The classic substitute for your own bone is someone else's bone obtained from a bone bank (banked bone or allograft bone; your own bone is called autograft bone).

Banked bone has received a bad reputation in the United States because of the news of two patients who contracted HIV from it. The cases were the result of totally unacceptable tissue-banking practices. With modern tissue-banking practices, developed for the most part in our world-renowned University of Miami Tissue Bank, the risks of developing a disease after receiving banked bone are fewer than the risks from receiving your own bone! The risks from taking your own bone include infection, fracture of the graft site, bleeding, and other risks. I am not aware of a reported case of a disease transmitted from banked bone grafts obtained from a qualified U.S. FDA–certified bone bank.

Banked bone has been shown to be as effective in obtaining a solid spinal fusion as your own bone, although the rate of fusion is slower with banked bone. The advantage of using banked bone over your own bone is that the surgery is faster, there is less blood loss, and you can use as much bone as is required. The quality of the bone may be better than your own bone, depending on your age and health status. The cost of banked bone is about the same as your own bone when you factor in the surgical cost of obtaining the bone graft from your pelvis. Consideration of the cost of grafts for spinal fusion is important when you consider the many bone-graft substitutes that are now available.

The most high-tech of the bone graft substitutes is genetically engineered bone morphogenic protein (BMP), a naturally occurring protein in your body that stimulates new bone formation. Genetically engineered BMP is now available for spinal fusion. It is as effective in producing a spinal fusion as your own bone. The big problem with it is that it costs more than $4,000 per spine level fused, compared to approximately $300 per level fused with your own bone or banked bone.

How do you know whether to fuse the spine from the back or from the front?

Spinal fusion is performed in three major ways. The most common way is by placing bone graft from behind on both sides between the transverse processes (bones that project to the sides of the boney arches behind each vertebra). This is called a posterior lateral fusion (see illustration page 84). The second way to perform a fusion is to place blocks of bone between the vertebrae themselves from behind, called a posterior interbody fusion. This type of fusion is only performed in the lumbar spine (see illustration page 86). The third type of fusion is performed by approaching the spine from the front and placing bone blocks between the vertebrae (anterior interbody fusion). This is the most common way to perform a fusion in the neck. Fusions from in front require removing the disc between the vertebrae and replacing it with a block of bone or a hollow metal cage filled with crushed bone or a sponge with genetically engineered BMP. The combination of a metal bone cage and BMP is very expensive, as you can imagine (more than $7,000 per level fused). Blocks of banked bone work just as well to maintain the space between the vertebrae and fuse them together, and they are a lot less expensive ($600 per level fused). Banked bone blocks have the additional advantage of having the same consistency as your vertebrae. The metal cages are too stiff, and it has been shown that they do not give as much pain relief as banked bone blocks.

Spinal fusions performed from behind require an incision over your spine, be it neck, chest, or low back, depending on where the fusion is indicated. Fusions between the vertebrae of your low back require an incision on your belly. To perform a fusion from in front of your thoracic spine requires an incision between the ribs adjacent to the level that is to be fused. And an intervertebral fusion in the neck requires an incision in front of the neck alongside your windpipe (trachea).

The type of fusion required to relieve your pain depends on many variables. The decision to fuse your spine with or without metal fixation, the type of bone graft to use, and the approach from behind or from in front should be made by a spinal surgeon based upon your circumstances. However, the decision to have your spine fused must be yours and yours alone. I show my patients their MRI scan and x-rays and explain what I think is needed to alleviate their painful condition. I specifically explain to them the need for metal fixation and the type of bone graft that I recommend. I explain the nature, benefits, and risks of the proposed surgery and answer all of their questions. The most frequently asked question is, "What would you do for your family member or yourself given my situation?" I affirm that what I am recommending to them is what I would personally have done if it were my back. I also tell them that, given the information that I have told them about the procedure, they must be the one to make the final decision to proceed. This process is called shared decision making, where the patient has all the facts from the doctor concerning the proposed surgery and makes their own decision based on those facts about whether to proceed with surgery.

You have undoubtedly noticed that I have discussed spinal fusion in conjunction with the deformities of the spine — spondylolisthesis, scoliosis, and kyphosis. No one can argue that spinal fusion is indicated when these conditions are the cause of or are contributing to your back pain. Intuitively it makes sense that if your spine is slipped, crooked, or bent over beyond the point of no return, something needs to be done to correct the deformity and stop it from getting worse. Why then the controversy over spinal fusion that you have read in the news?

Actually, there is evidence that too many spinal fusions are being performed. It is based upon population studies that show a wide regional variation in numbers of spinal fusions performed in North America. No one knows how many spinal fusions per capita is the appropriate number. But it is obvious that in some areas of North America too few people have this procedure and in some areas too many spinal fusions are being performed. Although healthcare planners and economists will eventually determine what the correct average number should be, that number still won't mean anything to you. What matters is whether a spinal fusion is the right thing for you or whether it is unnecessary in your case. The only way to determine this is to find a qualified spinal surgeon who will take the time to thoroughly explain your situation to you and let you decide what is best for you.

In my opinion, the reason that spinal fusion has received a bad name and is controversial is that it has been used too often to treat chronic "discogenic" low-back pain. I will discuss this issue in more detail in the next chapter on chronic discogenic back pain.

CHAPTER 8

Chronic Back Pain: What To Do When the Pain Just Won't Go Away

Most people (like my father) who suffer from acute attacks of back pain usually end up treating themselves. In most cases, that's perfectly all right. In between infrequent attacks they have little or no pain. The usual treatment is a short course of bed rest, anti-inflammatory medication, ice or heating pad, massage, and walking it off. These simple measures work for the vast majority of people. But what if your pain never really goes away? What if the attacks of severe pain keep recurring at shorter intervals? What if back pain is ruling your life? What then?

Why has the pain lasted so long? Is it from cancer?

If you have suffered from constant or recurring episodes of back pain for more than three months, then you have chronic back pain. Disc degeneration is the underlying cause of chronic back pain when it results in disc herniation, spinal stenosis, or spinal deformity. But what if these conditions are not the cause of your pain? What if your doctor has not been able to pinpoint why your back pain is lingering on? What if all kinds of treatment have been unsuccessful? What do you do now?

Your first priority is to find out what is really wrong. Make sure your doctor has exhausted all diagnostic tests that are necessary. I frequently see patients with MRI scans (see section on MRI starting on page 52) that have been performed in an open scanner that are so unclear that they need to be repeated in a closed scanner. On repeating the MRI in a closed scanner, I can often detect a subtle area of nerve entrapment that explains the patient's chronic back and leg pain.

I try to determine the characteristic of the pain. Is it neurogenic, from nerve entrapment; is it mechanical, from instability of the spine; is it arthritic, from facet joint arthritis, or is it discogenic, from the disc itself, (see Chapter 1)?

It may require that you have an injection of an MRI contrast dye with the scan to detect some painful conditions. Slow-growing tumors of the spinal nerves that cause progressively severe night pain and sleep disturbance can sometimes only be detected with a contrast-enhanced MRI scan. Good-quality MRI scans are very accurate in detection of most conditions that cause chronic back pain.

Another test that is used to detect low-grade infections, arthritic conditions, and tumors that may be the cause of chronic pain is a bone scan. This test is performed by injecting a short-acting radioactive chemical called Technesium into your vein, where it is taken up by the active bone-forming cells in your skeleton. You are then placed in a Geiger counter-type scanner that detects the radioactivity and turns it into a picture of your skeleton. If the bone-forming cells in your body are reacting to inflammation from arthritis, infection, or a tumor, a dark spot will show up in the picture of your skeleton. Some bone tumors (multiple myeloma, a cancer of the bone marrow) will inhibit bone-forming cells, which will appear as a hole in the skeleton on the bone scan.

This test is useful in detecting some chronically painful conditions of the spine. One of my sons could not play soccer because of chronic low-back pain localized to one side of his spine. He was in the middle of his growth spurt, played soccer for his high school team, and was lifting weights as most young men do at that age. He could not stand on one leg and lean backward without experiencing the pain. I suspected that he had a stress fracture of one of his pars interarticularis (see page 87), a common cause of chronic back pain in growing athletes who are required to hyperextend their back (lean backward) while playing their sport. Gymnasts, soccer players, golfers, tennis players, and football linemen are susceptible to this type of stress fracture of the spine.

My son's x-rays and MRI scan did not show the problem, but a bone scan pinpointed a stress fracture in his pars. I explained the problem to him and told him it would require at least seven months of not playing soccer or weight lifting to alleviate his pain. I did not advise him to wear a back brace, which was a common treatment for this condition at the time, because most young athletes will not wear one even if it is prescribed by the doctor. He listened to my advice, and he stayed in shape by swimming and bicycling exercises, both of which can be performed in flexion so as to keep stress off of the stress fracture. His pain went away in seven months and he was able to resume playing soccer for the remainder of his high school career.

Do I have arthritis?

There are several types of arthritis of the spine that can cause chronic generalized spine pain, one of which is ankylosing spondylitis (bone-forming inflammation of the spine), an inherited type of arthritis. The symptoms of ankylosing spondylitis (AS) first begin in young men (but rarely women) and are characterized by night pain and a feeling of stiffness on first arising in the morning. At first this disease is hard to diagnose, but later it becomes painfully apparent because it causes the spine to become bent forward (kyphosis). You may have seen someone with this condition walking on the street, bent over so far that it was difficult for them to see where they were going.

A bone scan and a blood test can detect this disease in its early stages and alert your doctor to begin treatment with anti-inflammatory medications and exercises to help ward off the deformity. Unfortunately in some cases the deformity occurs in the late stages of the disease despite the best treatment. In these cases the bent-forward spine can be straightened with surgery, which has become more effective with the use of pedicle screws.

Chronic pain that awakens you every night is serious and requires a specific diagnosis. If you can sleep in certain positions, e.g., on your side with your legs curled, you probably have spinal stenosis. But if you have to get up and walk around to relieve the pain and the pain is gradually getting worse each night, then you should question the possibility of a tumor (see page 26). Tumors may arise from the nerves in your spine or from the bone. The bad news is that breast and prostate cancer can metastasize to the vertebrae in your spine and cause chronic back pain. The good news is that most chronic back pain is not cancer, but is instead the consequence of one or more degenerated discs in your back.

Chronic discogenic back pain (degenerative disc disease)

The most common cause of chronic back pain stems from overzealous attempts at treating discogenic low-back pain, which is pain coming from the degenerated discs. Yes, that is correct – the treatment of discogenic pain may become part of the problem! Not a clinic day goes by that I do not see a patient who has a story that goes like this: "I have had this pain for so long that it's controlling my life. I have tried chiropractic, pain management, epidurals, acupuncture, you name it, and nothing seems to help." They are usually taking some combination of narcotics, muscle relaxants, and anti-inflammatory medications. They are depressed, can't sleep normally, and their whole world is falling apart around them. They have seen numerous different doctors and had numerous diagnostic tests. They say, "No one can find out what is wrong with me," or, even more ominously, "I have been told I need a fusion."

On delving into their problem further, I usually find something along these lines: initially they had an acute attack of back pain that was treated with a narcotic and a muscle relaxant; they were in bed for more than a few days; the pain did not get better, so they went to a chiropractor, whose treatments helped at first, so they kept going on a frequent basis so the pain would not come back. Eventually the pain returned, so they had an MRI scan which showed one or more degenerative dark disc(s); they were told they had a herniated disc and were referred to a pain-management specialist for a series of epidurals (see page 58). So, they were treated with more bed rest, physical therapy, acupuncture, traction, change of bed, corset, brace, facet injections, and intradiscal radiofrequency therapy (more about these in Chapter 9), but the pain still continued. When they finish telling me all of this, they are in tears and at their wits' end. They are convinced that something is drastically wrong because nothing has helped despite having spent thousands of dollars for health care.

Obtaining an accurate history from a patient who is suffering from chronic back pain is one of the most difficult tasks that I do. I have found that the best way to get to the bottom of the patient's problem is to listen until they finish telling their story without interrupting them. That is a very difficult thing for us doctors to do, because we immediately want to get to the bottom of the problem. We try to hurry up the process by interrupting just when you are getting to what is really troubling you. Try to tell your doctor exactly what you are thinking and the questions you want answered. Make sure your doctor answers these questions. This is very important when it comes to finding a solution to your chronic back pain.

After taking a thorough history from my patients, I perform a thorough physical examination. (Remember my aunt's story? She went to numerous doctors and no one examined her to determine she had pressure on her spinal cord that was causing her chronic pain.) Then I look at all of the patient's previously performed tests, x-rays, MRIs, CAT scans, etc. I get new tests if they are outdated or of poor quality (open MRI, see page 54), or if an essential test has not been performed. Once I am satisfied that the chronic pain is coming from degenerative disc disease, I explain this to my patient and reassure them that they have a good prognosis to be cured!

At this stage I try to determine whether they are significantly depressed. Most patients who have been taking narcotics and/or muscle relaxants for their pain for more than two weeks have some component of depression. If they had a predisposition to depression before they developed back pain, then pain medications may make it worse.

What roles do depression and stress have in my pain?

Depression accentuates chronic pain, and chronic pain accentuates depression. I have found that people who suffer from chronic pain almost always have significant depression. It brings to mind the question "which came first, the chicken or the egg?" It is important to know, because if the depression is the result of the treatment and pain, then discontinuing the pain medication, thus breaking the pain cycle, can resolve the depression and help alleviate the pain. But if the patient suffered from depression before the chronic back pain, they may require treatment with anti-depressant medication in order to obtain relief. If the patient has a PCP who knows them well, I work with that doctor to sort these issues out. If not, then I recommend a comprehensive pain rehabilitation center (more about them later).

I then explain to the patient that the key to their cure is to stop seeing doctors and stop all treatment for their pain except what they can do for themselves! At first this is a hard sell, so I explain to them that nothing has worked thus far to relieve their pain, therefore what do they have to lose by trying my approach? I explain that the pain will not get worse when they stop pain medication; in fact, they will feel better as soon as their own body's painkillers (endorphins) take over.

How can I get control of the pain and stop it from controlling me?

In order to stimulate their own body's painkillers, I tell them to walk a little more each day. Exercise is known to increase the endorphins in your body. The first day they should walk as far as the pain and their stamina will permit. I tell them not to be afraid of the pain, that it will not harm them even though it hurts. If they cannot tolerate walking I tell them to use a treadmill, stationary bicycle, or pool (aquatic) exercises. Any form of aerobic exercise is good, but it must be done every day. The goal is to build up to an hour a day of aerobic exercise (more about exercise for back pain in Chapter 9). If they smoke I advise them to stop right away and to lose weight or gain weight, whichever is appropriate for them. I tell them that this approach to their pain will not kill them, but continuing the treatment that they are getting might! My approach to chronic pain is safe and affordable. I reassure them that I will follow them in my clinic as frequently as they want and as long as it takes for their pain to subside. I also tell them that they can expect to have a markedly improved quality of life within three months of trying this approach. I tell them that if they do not have significant relief of their pain within three months, despite trying, we will perform new tests to determine what is wrong. This later advice is to reassure them, but it is rarely necessary because the majority of these patients are significantly improved by the end of three months. I also tell them that if their pain is not improved by these measures (no more treatments, no smoking, weight control, and exercise), and if it is determined that they would benefit from surgery, then it will be safe to have the surgery. Following this discussion most patients are extremely relieved and grateful. These are the patients who I know will be able to cure themselves of their chronic back pain.

It has been my observation that most patients who suffer from chronic discogenic back pain will obtain relief from the program that I described above. There is a well-designed study in the medical literature that supports this observation. The authors randomized people who suffered from chronic back pain into three treatment groups. One group was prescribed the usual physical therapy modalities of massage, ultrasound, and stretching. The second group was prescribed a moderate exercise program, and the third group more vigorous exercises. Within a three-month period, both exercise groups had significant relief of their chronic pain compared to the traditional physical therapy group. The results of this study are at first counterintuitive. You would at first think that more exercise would lead to more pain.

If you think back to the first chapter in this book, it will help you understand why exercise works. Recall that the disc is a living structure with living cells that depend on physical activity to live. When you walk around, water is squeezed out of the disc, and when you lie down the water is absorbed back into your disc. The flow of nutrients into and waste out of your discs keeps the cells healthy and allows them to keep your discs in repair. Lack of exercise and smoking kill the cells in your discs and cause them to become painful. It makes sense that controlled aerobic exercises will improve the health of the discs in your back and make them less painful.

The second reason my regime works is that it is aimed at restoring your own body's painkillers, endorphins, instead of depending on drugs that depress your endorphins and lead to mental depression, both of which increase your pain.

In the next chapter I will discuss most of the proven and unproven therapies out there for back pain. I will also describe the treatments that I have found to consistently work for my patients, the rationale behind them, their nature, benefits, risks, and costs.

CHAPTER 9

A Plethora of Back-Pain Care: Pills, Exercise, Injections, and Alternative Treatments

Every time I think that I have finally heard of all of the treatments foisted on the public for back pain, another one comes along. Recently a patient asked me about "astronaut chambers for back pain." It seems she had read an advertisement for this and was curious about my opinion of the treatment. I had to suppress a smile and formulate a hopefully intelligible answer at the same time. I asked her to send me the advertisement so that I could try to determine the rationale for this approach. Invariably patients will show me infomercials on the back-pain cure du jour. They ask me for my opinion concerning some new treatment that I have never heard of. I am usually suspicious of these treatments, since I have not seen or heard any qualified medical evidence to support the claims of their efficacy or safety. I should have come across something about them since I am on the editorial board of four medical journals and a member of 10 professional societies, all of which

I will tell you throughout this chapter what I think works and what to avoid in the way of treatment for your back pain.

evaluate new treatments on a regular basis. I will discuss some of these treatments if they are widely advertised, used, of historical interest, or new on the horizon. I will also discuss the theoretical basis and any evidence that is available in the medical literature to support or debunk their use.

In this chapter I will review the nature, benefits, risks, and costs of most of the back-pain treatments that I have heard of. I am positive I will miss a few, since new treatments for back pain appear on TV on a daily basis. Even on the way to work this morning I heard a so-called "public announcement" on NPR radio for minimally invasive spine surgery. I have organized this chapter into categories of treatments such as commonly prescribed medications, physical medicine modalities, injection therapies, pain management, and alternative treatments for back pain.

Throughout this book I have given you my approach to treatment of back pain. I will tell you throughout this chapter what I think works and what to avoid in the way of treatment for your back pain. But first, let's take a look at how the medical community evaluates the effectiveness of a particular treatment.

What is evidence-based medicine?

Evidence-based medicine is the process through which the medical community determines the effectiveness and safety of a treatment, with that determination being based on four different levels of evidence.

Level I evidence is derived from the results of well-designed clinical trials. This usually means a prospective, randomized, placebo-controlled study. A systematic review, meta-analysis, of a large number of peer-reviewed publications on a treatment also qualifies as Level I evidence.

Level II evidence means that there is at least one well-designed study or that multiple low-quality clinical trials have been reviewed.

Level III data comes from case series, studies not using placebo controls, and studies that compare results to historical controls.

Level IV studies are comparisons of multiple case series from different institutions.

The evidence-based effectiveness of a medication does not guarantee its availability. For example, chymopapain (chymo), an enzyme from the papaya fruit, was widely used throughout the world to dissolve herniated discs. There were three prospective, randomized, double-blind studies (neither the patient nor the doctor knew whether chymo or a placebo was being injected) from three countries that showed chymo was better than placebo to treat disc herniations. There were also several meta-analyses that showed the safety and efficacy of this treatment.

This was strong Level I evidence to support the use of chymopapain! Some of my most satisfied patients were those whom I treated with chymopapain for their disc herniations. Despite strong proof that chymo works, it is no longer available in North America. Why? Approximately 3,000 vials of chymopapain were sold per year in the United States, at $1,500/vial, for a total of $4.5 million revenue for the manufacturer. This revenue didn't even cover the liability insurance, let alone the production cost. Consequently the manufacturer stopped selling chymopapain in the United States in the early 1990s. Therefore a proven, safe, and effective method of treating herniated discs without surgery is no longer available. The same problem of liability cost has prevented an adequate supply of flu vaccines in the United States in the past.

Pills for back pain

The most commonly prescribed pills for back pain are anti-inflammatories, narcotics, and muscle relaxants. Over-the-counter anti-inflammatory pain medications work the best, are the safest and the least expensive of all the pills that are available for back pain. Ibuprofen (Advil) and naproxen (Aleve) are the two most popular over-the-counter anti-inflammatory medications. Like all anti-inflammatory medication, they can cause bruising, indigestion, heartburn, and gastrointestinal (GI) bleeding. They can also cause fluid retention with leg swelling. This can lead to elevation of blood pressure. People with kidney disease should not take these medications.

The anti-inflammatory effect of aspirin is the gold standard against which all others are measured. As good as aspirin is in relieving musculoskeletal pain, it has the major disadvantage of causing gastritis and GI bleeding. Most men whom I see are taking a baby aspirin, 81 mg/daily, as a preventative measure against a heart attack. It is useful for this because it inhibits blood clotting. Most people who do not have a pre-disposition to stomach upset can tolerate this low dose. However, between two and six aspirin a day (up to 1,800 mg) is needed for relief of back pain. These high doses of aspirin can cause life-threatening gastrointestinal bleeding, which is obviously a big risk to take for relief from benign back pain!

In my father's day, aspirin was the only anti-inflammatory medicine available. Although aspirin gave him relief from his back pain, he did complain that it caused him to have heartburn. To the best of my knowledge he never had any GI bleeding from it, but he did not take it very often, and when he did it was for a short period of time. Ibuprofen and naproxen are safer than aspirin with respect to GI bleeding, and they work as well as aspirin to relieve back pain. I do not recommend that you take aspirin for back pain. Nor do I recommend that you take any anti-inflammatory medication in large daily doses, or for more than a few days at a time.

The COX-2 inhibitors, Vioxx, Bextra, and Celebrex, are anti-inflammatory medications that were designed to give you pain relief without causing bleeding or indigestion. They do not irritate your stomach or cause bleeding as often as the anti-inflammatory medications mentioned above (the non–COX-2 inhibitors). When Vioxx was given on a daily basis for more than one year to a group of patients it was associated with close to a 4 percent incidence of heart attack or stroke compared to a 2 percent incidence of these events in an equivalent group of individuals taking a placebo. For this reason Vioxx, and subsequently Bextra, were taken off the market by their manufacturers. Celebrex is still available but is far less popular than it was before these findings were made public.

COX-2 anti-inflammatory medication like Celebrex requires a doctor's prescription and is expensive compared to over-the-counter anti-inflammatory medications. However, its advantages are that you only require one pill per day for effective relief of back pain and it can be used prior to spine surgery since it does not cause bleeding.

The anti-inflammatory drugs available to you today are safer than aspirin. However, I tell all of my patients not to take any anti-inflammatory medication on a daily basis. I tell them to take the medication one or two days in a row at the most. If they get relief, do not take them again unless the symptoms come back. No matter what, they should allow a one- or two-day interval between taking these pills to give their stomach a rest. If you develop heartburn or indigestion with any medication, stop it immediately. Also stop taking the medication if you develop black stools, which may mean stomach and intestinal bleeding.

The most potent of the anti-inflammatory pills that you can take are steroids. I discussed the benefits and risks of a short course of high-dose steroids (Medrol Dose-Pacs) in Chapter 3. I do not recommend steroids because there is not a good clinical study to prove that they are any better than your body's ability to relieve the pain on its own, and they have so many potentially serious side effects. A good prospective, randomized study of oral steroids versus placebo for the treatment of acute low-back pain and sciatica would show whether steroids are worth the risk. President Kennedy was treated with steroids for chronic low-back pain when he was a young man, with serious consequences! He was given too much steroid medication over too long of a time period, which caused his adrenal glands (the glands that produce your own body's steroids) to permanently stop functioning. This resulted in a condition that requires that you take steroids the rest of your life. If you do not take them, you develop symptoms that can be life threatening. Granted, today doctors are aware that too much steroid can cause this complication, and this is the reason why safe dosage schedules where developed (Dose-pacs), but I still see patients who have been treated with more than one series of steroids who are in danger of developing a dependency on steroids similar to that which plagued President Kennedy for much of his life.

Acetaminophen (Tylenol) is the most popular over-the-counter non-narcotic pain medication in North America. It does not irritate your stomach and does not cause bleeding. However, too much Tylenol can cause liver damage. Also, if you are known to have liver disease, history of hepatitis, or drink heavily you should not take acetaminophen. I do not recommend to my patients that they take more than six Tylenol daily (total daily dose of 1,800 mg). And I do not recommend that they take it on a daily basis.

Narcotic pain medication must be prescribed by a physician. The most prescribed narcotic painkillers in North America are, in increasing order of potency: Codeine, Tylenol with Codeine, Darvocet, Percocet, Morphine, Vicoden, Dilaudid, Oxycontin, Oxycodone, and Methadone. They are highly effective for relief of acute pain, such as post-operative pain. The big problem with narcotics is that they deplete the body's natural painkillers (endorphins) within your body. This begins to happen within three or four days of taking them. When your endorphins are depleted you become depressed, and this in turn causes you to suffer more from your pain. Also, narcotics make you drowsy, impair your driving skills, and are constipating. Narcotics make some people become hyper. Since most back-pain conditions are relatively benign (not cancer), tend to last more than three days and recur frequently, and narcotics have so many side effects when taken for more than a few days, I do not recommend them to my patients for chronic back pain. On the contrary, I try to take patients suffering from chronic back pain off of narcotics when I think that they are contributing to the suffering. The objective of this approach is to relieve their suffering from chronic pain and improve their quality of life.

Most oral narcotics are not habituating, so people do not become dependent on them. That is, you can rapidly wean yourself off of them without having withdrawal symptoms. However, strong narcotics such as Oxycontin, Methadone, Fentanyl, and Dilaudid are the exception. I have observed that patients who are taking these potent narcotics require escalating doses of them to obtain relief of pain, become depressed and dependent on them, and they have withdrawal symptoms when they stop taking these drugs. For these reasons I do not ever prescribe potent narcotics to my patients, except in the immediate post-operative period. I have also found that the patients I see who are taking these drugs for chronic back pain are still complaining of their pain, therefore the pain medication is not working anyway! In fact, the pain medication has become one of the primary causes of the pain in some patients, and lasting pain relief depends on stopping them. It is difficult to explain this to patients who have chronic pain that is enhanced by the painkillers that they depend on for relief. Some patients will not believe this explanation and will continue to suffer from chronic pain. I have never seen a patient who requires a large amount of narcotics for chronic back pain obtain satisfactory relief and a good quality of life. However, I have seen numerous patients with chronic back pain who have been cured by being weaned off of narcotics!

Muscle relaxants fall into the same category as potent narcotics when it comes to causing depression and enhancing chronic pain. Muscle relaxants lead to depression, are habituating, and it is difficult to stop taking them. Patients frequently tell me that they were previously prescribed a muscle relaxant that they stopped taking because it made them drowsy and did not relieve the pain anyway. If you have been taking Valium or other potent muscle relaxants for an extended period of time, you must be weaned off of them slowly, over a period of time. A too-rapid withdrawal of these medications can lead to seizures, so you should ask your doctor to give you a safe schedule for stopping them. I do not recommend muscle relaxants to my patients for relief of chronic back pain. However, I will prescribe one dose of Valium to my claustrophobic patients to help them get through an MRI scan because it makes them less aware of what is happening and thereby relieves their claustrophobia.

Two frequently prescribed medications for neurogenic back pain are Neurontin (the generic form is Gabapentin) and Lyrica. They are commonly prescribed for chronic nerve pain as an off-label use (use of a drug for a purpose other than what it was approved for). Gabapentin is a U.S. FDA–approved anti-seizure medication. Neurologists (specialists in diseases of the nervous system, brain, spinal cord, and nerves, see page 40) have also found it to be useful in treating abnormal sensations experienced from peripheral neuropathy (a disease of the nerves that causes annoying sensations in the lower legs, usually seen in diabetics). They then began using it for patients with chronic nerve pain from spinal stenosis. Like some narcotics and muscle relaxants, it causes drowsiness and it must be withdrawn slowly. Many patients have told me that the side effects of this drug are not worth the relief it gives them. I prescribe these for some patients with neurogenic pain (see Chapter 6), but most of the time I wean patients off of these drugs because they are not helping to alleviate the symptoms for which they were being prescribed.

Pain-management specialists frequently prescribe slow-release skin patches containing narcotics (Fentanyl) and local anesthetics (Lidoderm) for chronic back pain. I find that it is very difficult for patients to wean themselves off of Fentanyl patches, a potent narcotic that is quite addictive. Lidoderm patches are not addicting, and I find they are useful for some patients with nerve pain. Lidoderm patches can only be used for 12 hours at a time, and I prescribe them for patients who are having difficulty sleeping because of nerve pain in the legs or arms. I think they should only be used for acute pain and for a short period of time.

Physical medicine, rehabilitation, and modalities for back pain

We will look at ridiculous things like "astronaut chambers" and hanging traction to physical methods that have been proven through evidence-based medicine, such as aerobic exercise and some forms of traction. I will then recommend the physical treatments that I have seen help my patients. Physical methods of treatment include immobilization in corsets or braces, chiropractic, massage, electrical stimulation, physical therapy, heat and ice, acupuncture, TENS (transcutaneous electrical nerve stimulation) traction, manipulation, and trigger-point acu-pressure.

One person swears by chiropractic, the other says it's quackery. Which is it?

I have studied the chiropractic method and used this method to treat selected patients throughout the years. Chiropractic has a place in relieving certain painful conditions of the spine, especially acute back pain in young adults. However, there are some older patients for whom the method should not be used, which I will explain later. Like other treatments for back pain, such as medications and surgery, it tends to be overused. Here is how I use chiropractic and when I think it should not be used.

The most common treatment people have for back pain today is chiropractic. I have used this method to treat patients over the years and have observed many patients who claim to have benefited from it prior to seeing me. I have also seen a number of patients who complain that their herniated disc was caused by a chiropractic adjustment. The objective of chiropractic is to relieve back pain by realigning the spine using manipulation.

The manipulations may be any combination of stretching, twisting, or bending your spine by the chiropractor in so-called "adjustments."

I have helped a number of patients over the years with a manipulation in an acute episode of back pain. I learned this treatment in the early years of my practice from a qualified practitioner. I was also invited to be the keynote speaker by the American Chiropractic Association at one of its annual meetings. It was at Disney World in Orlando shortly after it opened. My four children were very young at the time and they still remember the four days we stayed at the Contemporary Hotel inside the park because of the monorail that runs through the hotel. I presented six hours of lectures on how to determine which patients should not be manipulated. The lectures were well attended and received. Since then I have maintained a good relationship with the chiropractic profession, which has been of benefit to all of our patients.

To illustrate how I have used the chiropractic method I will tell you of several instances in which it helped people. I received a call from one of my neighbors who, while lifting a large potted plant on his patio, experienced severe low-back pain. He was lying on the floor when I arrived. He is over six-feet seven-inches tall, a former professional basketball player, and is one of the happiest and most loquacious individuals I have ever met. He informed me straight off that his pain was no joke! After reassuring myself that he did not have a serious problem, I helped him to stand up and performed a standing traction type of manipulation, which helped to straighten him. He had immediate relief from back pain. For months after this episode he would vocally proclaim my skill in every crowded venue where we would meet. How embarrassing! Had I known he would do this I never would have manipulated his back...just kidding, neighbor!

Another episode that comes to mind to illustrate the usefulness of a manipulation occurred many years ago. A colleague called me to see one of his patients between my surgical cases. It turned out that the lady had come from her winter home in the Bahamas in her own private plane just to have a manipulation to ease her neck pain. I saw her in an examining room alongside the operating room between my surgical cases and determined that she was a good candidate for a manipulation and performed the procedure. She had immediate relief, was grateful, and I went back to surgery. I had totally forgotten the episode when, several months later, I ran into my colleague in the courtyard of our medical center. He said that he had been carrying around a thank-you note from the lady and handed it to me. I put it in my white coat pocket and went about my business. Some time later, when I was emptying my coat pocket, I came across the note and opened it. It was a very gracious thank-you note, and attached to the note was a generous contribution to my research fund! Needless to say, I was surprised.

My son kept telling me about his friend's mother, who had been back and forth to the hospital for chest pain. At first the doctors thought that she was having a heart attack, but all her test results were normal. She must have suffered for six months before she came to see me with pain in one area of her thoracic spine. I examined her and reviewed all of her x-rays and concluded that the pain was coming from her spine and that it was not from something serious like cancer or an infection. As I was giving her a spinal manipulation we both heard a popping sound in her back, and her pain was cured. Although there is no way to prove it, I think the manipulation straightened a misaligned joint between one of her ribs and the adjacent vertebrae. Of course my son then spread this story around the neighborhood, and I was the local hero for having cured her pain after she had suffered for so many months.

The problem with chiropractic treatment is illustrated by the following episode. It is difficult to determine who is a good candidate for chiropractic, whom it would be dangerous to perform it on, and exactly what is taking place when it is performed that relieves the pain.

My late friend, medical partner, and neighbor, who ran several miles daily to keep in shape, would suffer from periodic episodes of benign low-back pain. During these attacks he would lean to one side like the Leaning Tower of Pisa. I treated him with spinal manipulation on more than one occasion, but I was not convinced it did much to shorten his course of pain or to relieve it to any degree. He was not sure either, so we stopped doing it after a few attempts. The point about this case is that if it does not work with a few tries, quit having it done.

When should I have chiropractic, and when should I avoid it?

The point of all of these stories is that a manipulation can help relieve acute neck, chest, and low-back pain in the right candidate, but *not* in older people, not sick people, and not people who have had an injury. There is no place for it in chronic back pain, in my opinion. In fact, repeated manipulations over an extended period of time may contribute to chronic pain (more about this in Chapter 8).

My father may have benefited from chiropractic manipulation for his acute attacks of back pain. On the other hand, my aunt could have been seriously harmed by a manipulation for her neck pain because she had a severe constriction of her spinal canal pressing on her spinal cord. A manipulation of her spine could have left her acutely paralyzed.

Your chiropractor is well aware of who is a candidate for adjustments and who should not have spinal adjustments. I only adjust patients after I am satisfied that they do not have a herniated disc, severe spinal stenosis, a vertebral fracture, osteoporosis, arthritis, an infection, or a tumor. Rarely will I perform a spinal manipulation on someone over 60 years of age, and I would not manipulate anyone under the age of 16. These are the age groups in which serious conditions are more likely to be causing the back pain.

There is some clinical research – evidence-based medicine – that shows that the natural course of acute low-back pain attacks can be shortened by manipulations. I have seen this in my patients and use this method when it is indicated.

Periodically I will see a patient who has gotten into the habit of repeatedly twisting their neck or low back for relief. I call this "auto-manipulation," and I do not advocate this. I think that repeated passive twisting of the spine must contribute to further weakening of a degenerated disc. Although the manipulation feels good at the time, it may result in more back pain a few days later when a sprained disc becomes inflamed and painful.

Another scenario I sometimes see is the person who had dramatic relief of an acute back pain by a chiropractic treatment. They are then convinced to have "maintenance treatments" to prevent further attacks of pain.

The manipulations are performed not only at the originally painful area of the spine, e.g., low back, but along the entire spine. The person then begins to develop aching along the whole spine but does not attribute these new symptoms to the repeated manipulations. When I see a patient with this history I suggest that they stop all treatments, and their generalized spine pain goes away. I have seen similar symptoms that have been caused by repeated deep massage or the use of a vibrating device. I suspect that the small joints in the spine – the paired facet joints at each disc level of the entire spine – are irritated by repeated manipulation or vibration and become symptomatic from these maneuvers. For this reason I do not recommend repeated manipulations, massage, or vibration for treatment of spine pain.

There are possible risks from manipulation of the spine, just as there are with any treatment. The most serious reported complications of spinal manipulation are stroke, paralysis, massive disc herniation with cauda equina syndrome (see page 30), and vertebral fracture. Degenerative disc disease in the neck usually results in the build-up of bone spurs (osteophytes) around the border of the disc. There is a pair of arteries (vertebral arteries) carrying blood to your brain in a tight bony canal on either side of the discs in your neck. These arteries can be constricted by bone spurs from adjacent degenerative discs. There have been cases in which a manipulation of the neck caused the bone spurs to block the arteries, causing a stroke, blindness, and even death. The same bone spurs can contribute to spinal stenosis in your neck. There have been case reports of paralysis coming from manipulation of an arthritic neck when the bone spurs were made to press harder into the spinal cord. I do not recommend that older individuals who are prone to degenerative arthritis have manipulation for pain because of these risks.

What about traction?

Literally, just as I was about to write this section my wife handed me an advertisement from the *Miami Herald*. "How Space Age Technology Is Solving Back Pain Without Drugs Or Surgery," complete with a toll-free number. I called, and the presumable inventor's recorded voice suggested

I leave my name and address and he would send me the information on this dramatic space-age cure. The ad listed a web page that provided the name of the device, which I immediately Googled. It turned out to be yet another iteration of a traction device to reduce herniated discs. The web page was cleverly designed with links to medical journals touting the efficacy of the device. One of the articles featured a pre- and post-treatment MRI scan that showed reduction of a lumbar disc herniation. The treatment requires that you spend 45 minutes a day for a minimum of two weeks on the traction machine to guarantee 86 percent good results! I have had patients tell me that this course of treatment cost them more than $3,000. In my experience, if they had walked the pain off for two weeks instead of undergoing this treatment, they would have had better than a 90 percent chance of "good results" without the expense. This is the type of cleverly presented information that often appears in advertisements and on websites, which you must try to interpret in an attempt to find a cure for back pain.

The rationale for traction treatments is that the normal disc height is restored and/or disc herniations are reduced, thus taking the pressure off of the nerves to relieve the pain. What seemed to be a well-designed medical study from Scandinavia showed that traction was more effective than waiting it out in cases of painful lumbar disc herniation. I had already seen many patients who had undergone hanging traction treatment for disc herniations and back pain in a center devoted to this treatment in Miami. The center did not last long. I was not impressed with their results and was not impressed with the results of the Scandinavian study either. I have seen several patients who were injured by hanging traction devices over the years. I think this is a potentially dangerous method of treatment, particularly for older individuals who are susceptible to stroke. I do not recommend this type of treatment for my patients.

From an anatomical standpoint, most symptomatic disc herniations occur when the central spongy part of the disc (nucleus pulposus) "button holes" through a hole in the outer rim of the disc (annulus fibrosus). When traction is placed on this type of disc herniation, the button hole tightens up and traps the displaced disc in the spinal canal. The traction has the effect of further stretching the nerve root over the disc herniation, which can result in more pain and nerve damage. I have talked to a number of patients who said that their leg pain was worse as the result of traction, and I suspect this is what happened to them.

I have seen patients who were suffering only from back pain who later also developed leg pain as the result of traction treatment. I suspect that a degenerated disc was actually herniated by the traction in these cases.

Neck traction can relieve acute severe arm pain from a herniated disc. There are neck-traction devices that you can use in your home that have been around for as long as I can remember. I have not prescribed them in recent years because they are cumbersome and it is difficult to teach patients how to use them. Also, the arm pain is relieved while you are hanging in the device, but it returns as soon as the traction is released. You cannot sit around all day long with your neck in traction. I find that patients get more relief from walking it off than they do sitting in traction.

What kind of exercise works? Should I stretch?

Exercise is very important for the treatment and prevention of acute and chronic back pain. In fact, I think it is one of the most effective things that you can do. There are several studies and observations that I have made to convince me that exercise is important. One study compared one group of people who were treated with two days of bed rest for acute low-back pain with another group who were treated with one week of bed rest. The people who were mobilized after two days had 46 percent fewer sick days, suffered less, and recovered more quickly. Another study looked at three groups of people who suffered from chronic low-back pain. One group was treated with vigorous exercise, a second group with mild exercise, and the third group with massage and other modalities. The vigorous exercise group had the best pain relief and return of function compared to the other two groups. The final study was performed on firefighters. Again, three groups were compared. The first group exercised vigorously every day. The second group exercised intermittently, and the third group did not exercise at all. Over a three-year period, the firefighters who exercised vigorously every day had significantly fewer and less severe attacks of back pain and lost less time from work than the other two groups. The best way to treat acute back pain is to walk it off (first study), and exercise is also the best way to treat chronic back pain (second study). In addition, exercise is the best way to prevent back pain (third study). I have found this to be true for my patients, and it's also what works for me!

There are three goals for exercise: strength, stamina, and flexibility. Flexibility is supposedly enhanced by stretching. There are a number of stretching programs touted for treatment of back pain. Yoga, McKenzie, and Pilates are the three most popular stretching exercises for back pain. Some forms of yoga and Pilates also build strength and stamina, whereas the program proposed by McKenzie is purely a stretching type of exercise. McKenzie advocates lying on your stomach and passively hyper-extending your back by pushing your body up with your arms. The theory is that this maneuver reduces the disc herniation and relieves pressure on the nerves. I personally have experienced an exacerbation of low-back pain a day or two after trying this type of stretching, which I think comes from irritation of my facet joints by this maneuver. I may not be a candidate for the McKenzie system, and I have not been able to determine who is. I definitely do not recommend passive hyper-extension of your back if you have spinal stenosis. This maneuver will make the stenosis worse and can exacerbate the pain. I am not an advocate of the McKenzie method.

The Pilates system is based on exercise equipment that passively stretches you as you actively strengthen your muscles. It was originally popularized as a method for rehabilitation of injured ballet dancers. It is probably a good system for high-performance entertainers who are young, agile, and require a controlled exercise system to stimulate rapid healing of sprained ligaments, but I am not sure that it is a good system for most back-pain sufferers. It requires that you be attended by a physical therapist who is familiar with the system. I have not recommended it to my patients because I do not think it is a good system for people suffering from degenerative diseases of the spine. I think it should be used to assist in the rehabilitation of the injured athletes for which Pilates designed the system.

I have developed the same prejudice against yoga for chronic back pain from degenerative disc disease. I have seen numerous patients over the years who have made their pain worse as the result of the passive rotary maneuvers performed in yoga. One patient actually developed a massive disc herniation with cauda equina syndrome from a yoga maneuver. However, I must admit that many patients extol the virtues of yoga for their well being and relief of back pain. I do not recommend the vigorous twisting maneuvers performed in yoga. It is also potentially harmful to your back if you are passively twisted or stretched by someone else during yoga.

Of the three components of exercise – strength, agility and stamina – which combination is the best for managing your back pain? As you may have gathered from my discussion of the passive stretching systems such as McKenzie and Pilates, I am not an advocate of these systems. It does not make sense to passively stretch an already-weakened degenerative disc. As the disc begins to degenerate, it becomes unstable. In the late stages of disc degeneration, reparative processes cause the disc to stiffen up again. As the disc becomes stiffer it becomes less susceptible to injury, but subjecting it to repeated stretching will prevent it from stiffening. For this reason I am not a fan of passive stretching for back pain as the result of disc degeneration.

Muscle-strengthening exercises are good for your back as long as you avoid lifting heavy weights through your spine. I have seen a few athletes who have blown out a degenerated disc through heavy weight lifting. I advise my patients to use the weight machines and do only bench presses, but not to snatch weights off of the floor or lift overhead. For people who are interested in keeping good muscle tone while they are getting over an attack of back pain (yes, there are people who want to do this), I suggest light weights and multiple repetitions for the arms and the quadriceps machines for the legs (the one in which you sit and straighten your legs against resistance). If you have back pain, do not do the hamstring muscle exercise in which you lie on your stomach and bend your knee against resistance. This maneuver tends to arch your back and can exacerbate your back pain. I am not an advocate of excessive muscle-strengthening exercises for back pain, but I do advocate keeping good muscle tone.

The most important exercises that you can do to relieve back pain and prevent it are those that improve your stamina. Walking outdoors or indoors on a treadmill, bicycle exercise, and aquatic exercises are the best aerobic exercises for your back. If you have acute or chronic back pain, do whichever one you can do within the limits of your pain and stamina.

Initially you may have to start out slowly doing aquatic pool exercises and gradually work up to walking an hour a day. This is what my wife and I do to keep fit and ward off back-pain attacks. These aerobic exercises not only strengthen your leg muscles, but they also strengthen the muscles around your entire spine. They also stimulate your own body's painkillers, your endorphins. Additionally, aerobic exercise has been shown to improve your balance, reflexes, and coordination, thus making you less susceptible to falling and injuring your back. All of these benefits of aerobic exercise help relieve back pain and prevent it from recurring. Aerobic exercise is the single most important thing you can do to make your back pain go away and keep it from coming back!

The following is an actual e-mail that I received from a former patient while I was writing this book, which I share with you with the sender's permission. She was in her mid-30s when I saw her for the first time and she suffered from chronic low-back pain from a severely degenerated disc. A spinal fusion or artificial disc replacement had been suggested to her before she consulted me. I recommended that she avoid twisting and passive stretching maneuvers and perform aerobic exercises instead of having a procedure performed on her spine. This is what she wrote:

> *Hi Dr. Brown,*
>
> *I just wanted to send you a quick note to say hello as well as give you a little update. I had seen you over a year ago and you had discovered that one of my discs had basically disintegrated. Although I was in a lot of constant pain, you gave me great advice on movements and exercises not to make and ever since then, my back has been fantastic! I am also 8 months pregnant and although many women complain of back problems during pregnancy, mine has been just fine.*
>
> *Thank you again for such sound medical advice – I can see why my brother-in-law raved about how you were the one who saved him from surgery after three other doctors said there was no alternative.*

I hope you and your family had a fantastic Thanksgiving weekend and wishing you the best through the Holiday season!

Best regards!
Tia

Every back-pain book or pamphlet has diagrams of specific exercises for the spine, some of which look harmful to your back under some circumstances. When I ask patients to demonstrate the exercises that they are doing, most of them show me maneuvers that are harmful to someone with a degenerated disc. The maneuvers that require leaning back, passive twisting, and rotation of the spine are the ones that concern me. A study was published recently that confirmed my impression that back-specific exercises are actually harmful to your back!

There is a well-designed prospective randomized study comparing the effect of back-specific exercises to low-stress recreational physical activity, such as walking and swimming, on acute and chronic back pain. The study found that back-specific exercises actually increased the likelihood of back pain and disability, whereas aerobic exercise decreased acute and chronic back pain, disability, and stress. People who perform the equivalent of three hours a week of brisk walking or similar aerobic exercise benefited from the most reduction in back pain, stress, and disability. It works for my family, my patients, and me, and it has been shown to work in several well-designed studies: consistent low-impact aerobic exercise is the best medicine for acute, recurring, and chronic back pain. The really good news is that you don't have to do those ridiculous back exercises (that are hard to learn, remember, and perform) to get relief and prevent future attacks of back and neck pain.

Do I need a physical therapist or trainer? How about pain management?

Whether you should exercise on your own or have physical therapy depends on how physically fit you are, and whether you can do it on your own or need help from a physical therapist or trainer.

How do you know if you are physically fit enough to do it on your own without a physical therapist?

People fall into roughly four categories of fitness. These categories are not age-dependent. My mother exercised every day of her life and remained physically fit into her 90s. She rarely complained of back pain, although I remember that she had a few attacks of neck pain when she was younger. She remained in the fit category her whole life and enjoyed a great quality of life up until the time she died at the age of 97. She clearly fit into the first category, which is comprised of people who are physically fit, perform aerobic exercise regularly, are of normal weight, and do not have not chronic aliments. They also do not drink excessively and do not smoke.

The second group does not exercise regularly, are not too heavy or too thin, do not drink heavily, and do not smoke. If they have a chronic disease, such as high blood pressure or diabetes, it is under control.

The third group of people is physically sedentary, overweight or too thin, may smoke and/or drink too much, and may be taking medications for pain. This group gets short of breath from walking up a flight of stairs.

The last group of people is deconditioned from inactivity and/or chronic disease and may require a walker or wheel chair to get around. They cannot walk up a flight of stairs.

If you are in the first group, it is very likely that you can walk off an acute attack of back pain with just the reassurance from your doctor that it is safe to do so. Most of my fit patients do this on their own.

If you are in the second group, you may need the help of a physical therapist for pain relief and assistance in how to exercise in the face of pain. Some patients can do it without a therapist and some cannot. A lot of it has to do with what they can afford and what their insurance will cover. I recommend physical therapy for acute back pain for patients who don't think they can do it on their own.

I recommend to people who are in the third category of fitness that they see their PCP to have a general medical examination. If they are over the age of 60 and/or have hypertension, diabetes, or a history of smoking, I suggest to their PCP that they have a non-treadmill cardiac stress test to be sure that their heart can tolerate an exercise program. I recommend a proper diet, no smoking, and no drinking. After I am assured that they can start an exercise program, I refer them to a physical therapist. Physical therapists teach, guide, and monitor them in the rehabilitation process.

After those who are in the fourth category have been examined by their PCP, I usually refer them to an inpatient comprehensive pain rehabilitation program where they have immediate access to multiple specialists including a physical therapist for pain control and rehabilitation. The inpatient setting is important because of the numerous problems this group of patients needs help with, i.e., diet, pain control, detoxification, conditioning, and other medical problems.

Group I
Physically Fit
When reassured by your doctor that it is safe,
"Walk it off" on your own.

Group 2
Good health but not physically fit
When reassured by your doctor that it is safe, consult a physical therapist for pain relief and how to exercise within the limits of pain and stamina.

Group 3
Poor health and/ or poor health habits
See your doctor for a cardiac stress test and treatment of chronic conditions, and when it is determined to be safe, consult a physical therapist to teach, guide, and monitor in the rehabilitation process.

Group 4
Physically debilitated
Inpatient comprehensive pain rehabilitation center.

What about pain management for my chronic back pain?

Pain management is a specialty in medicine that arose out of a need to provide a comprehensive approach to people who suffer from chronic pain from cancer, neurological diseases, arthritis, and musculoskeletal diseases such as chronic back pain. A comprehensive pain-management team may be comprised of anesthesiologists, physiatrists, neurologists, psychologists, nurses, and physical therapists. They manage pain medication, nerve blocks, epidural pumps, psychological care, and alternative approaches such as acupuncture.

In our community we have a world-renowned comprehensive pain rehabilitation center (CPRC) that offers inpatient as well as outpatient treatment for chronic pain. A CPRC offers similar specialties and services as a comprehensive pain management center with more emphasis on rehabilitation.

I recommend the CPRC approach to my debilitated chronic back pain patients. I frequently will refer patients to a pain management specialist for epidural injections for acute nerve pain from a herniated disc, but I prefer to manage their chronic pain myself. I believe it is in my patients' best interest to have quick pain relief for acute back pain conditions. I also do not want them to become dependent on treatment, so I always plan to initiate rehabilitation along with acute pain management right from the beginning, to prevent chronic pain syndromes from occurring. It has been my observation that pain management centers do not seem to be able to do this as well. I think it takes a one-to-one relationship with the patient to make my approach effective.

How about minimally invasive treatments?

What about other treatments, such as epidurals, radiofrequency ablation, Botox, sclerosing agents, cryoablation, Chymopapain, intradiscal radiofrequency therapy (IDET) for back pain? You can ask your doctor about these, but how does he or she determine what works and what is safe? I examine the evidence-based medicine (see page 108) for a specific treatment;

determine whether it makes sense, is safe, and if I would personally take the treatment. Then, I decide whether to recommend it to my patients.

Treating back pain by destroying sensory nerves

There is a class of treatments for back pain that is based upon killing the sensory nerves in your back. These nerves are responsible for sending pain sensation from the facet joints, ligaments, and discs in your back to your brain. The rationale for destroying these nerves is to stop the source of the pain. The first method to be developed in this class was facet rhizotomy, a method that uses a long, thin knife to cut the nerves to the facet joints. The method was the rage in Australia, which is where it was developed. It was soon apparent to Australian doctors that it did not work and was dangerous, so the procedure's popularity declined faster than its meteoric climb.

Coincidentally, as I was writing this section I received an e-mail requesting my opinion concerning what was the correct choice for a patient. The patient was in his 50s and was continuing to have pain following a micro-discectomy. One physician had recommended revision spine surgery and another had recommended an IDET procedure with a 75 percent chance of a good result. My reply was that IDET is a method of destroying the nerve endings in the peripheral layers of a painful disc to relieve back pain. The clinical studies show that it is a relatively safe procedure, but the results are not much better than letting the condition heal on its own. It is also an expensive procedure.

In addition to having the pain nerves in your back cut (rhizotomy) and burned (IDET), you can have them electrocuted (percutaneous facet rhizotomy), frozen (cryoablation), and now poisoned, no less, with Botox! Thankfully I have not heard of a method of hanging the nerve.

Electrocuting the nerves by percutaneous facet rhizotomy has been proven to be no better than placebo in a well-designed, controlled clinical trial. Botox has been shown to give short-term relief compared to placebo in a small trial. The procedure is rigorous, requiring multiple injections under fluoroscopy, is potentially dangerous and expensive, and I would not recommend it.

I do not mean to be facetious when discussing these various attempts at destroying the pain nerves in your facet joints or discs to relieve back pain, but none of them has passed rigorous Level I trials showing efficacy compared to placebo or long-term efficacy as determined by meta-analysis (page 108). I have not encountered people who have had these types of procedures who feel that they helped for a long period of time. I do not recommend any of them because of lack of efficacy, potential danger, and high cost.

I have already discussed the rationale for epidural steroid injections in the chapter on disc herniation. There is Level I evidence for the short-term efficacy and safety for the use of epidurals for disc herniation, but not for spinal stenosis. The majority of patients for whom I have prescribed epidurals have had enough pain relief from their disc herniation to be able to stop taking narcotics and sleep through the night. It is a relatively safe treatment, but it's expensive. I do not recommend more than three epidurals in a six-month period. I think that the lifetime total number of epidurals should be limited to six. Too many epidurals can lead to chronic holes in the dural sac containing the nerves and scarring around the nerves. If the nerve continues to be irritated after six epidural steroid injections, it is my opinion that you should consider surgery to relieve the impingement on the nerve.

Epidurals are administered in the middle of your back, where the steroid is injected into the epidural space in the central spinal canal at the level of the disc herniation. They can also be placed from the side into the channel through which a specific nerve is traveling, which is the trans-foraminal approach. Either way, they should be performed with the use of a fluoroscopy machine so that the doctor can see exactly where the injection is going. I think epidurals provide better and faster pain relief and are safer than giving steroids by mouth, although they are much more expensive than oral steroids (see page 58 for a complete description of epidural injections).

Are back braces ever useful?

Immobilization with corsets and braces has been an old-time mainstay for treatment of acute and chronic back pain. There is no data to authenticate their use. I find that older deconditioned individuals with a component of mechanical back pain from spondylolisthesis, vertebral fractures, and scoliosis seem to benefit from a corset or brace, and they are the only patients who will wear them. Some people find they are helpful in relieving acute attacks of low-back pain. I have gotten away from prescribing cervical collars for acute neck pain. I think patients actually get over acute attacks of neck pain sooner if they keep moving. When neck pain is preventing a person from getting to sleep, I do recommend a soft collar.

"Touch" therapy

There is a class of treatments in which stimulation of skin sensation through heat, ice, light touch, tickling, and vibration stimulates the release of your own painkillers, the endorphins. None of these methods will relieve pain if you are taking narcotics or muscle relaxants, because these medications deplete and block the action of your endorphins. Skin stimulation also works because the brain gives precedence to skin sensation over pain sensation from deep ligamentous structures like painful discs and facet joints. Acupuncture, Transcutaneous Neural Stimulation (TENS), Rolfing, and light massage are some of the modalities that fall into this category.

After two days of unaccustomed lifting and bending while cleaning up my yard after Hurricane Wilma, I experienced backache that was keeping me from falling asleep. My wife gave me *cosquillitas* (means "little tickles" in Spanish) on my back, and within a few minutes the backache and muscle spasm subsided and I was able to fall asleep. Don't laugh; try it sometime when you are having an attack of back pain. It really works! *Cosquillitas* work in the same way as acupuncture, and are arguably a lot less expensive, less painful, and more fun than getting stuck with acupuncture needles!

There are a lot of treatments out there from which to choose for your back pain. Most of them have not passed the test of Level I evidence-based medicine or the test of time. Some are safe, effective, and inexpensive, and you can do them yourself (aerobic exercise). Some are just the opposite: dangerous, ineffective, and expensive (facet rhizotomy), and should be avoided. Using the information I have given you in this chapter, you can access the Web and find out for yourself which treatments are good and which ones do not seem right. You should then discuss them with your doctor and find out what she or he thinks about the treatment and whether it is right for you.

CHAPTER 10

What You Can Do To Avoid 'Failed Back Syndrome'

Failed back syndrome (FBS) refers to persistent or recurrent symptoms following previous back surgery. The original surgery may have failed to relieve the pain, or it only relieved it for a period of time and then the original pain recurred, or a different pain occurred.

What is a failed back syndrome? Why does it happen? How do I get rid of it? How do I keep that from happening to me?

The most common reason for failed back syndrome

I have found that the most common reason for failed back-pain surgery is that the patient was not prepared for the original surgery before it was performed. People who are on high doses of painkillers and who are deconditioned will experience little relief from spine surgery for back pain. Because of this they are difficult to mobilize and impossible to rehabilitate following surgery. Often the original source of pain was magnified by the pain medication they were taking before surgery, and the surgical procedure made the pain even worse. I suspect that if these patients had been weaned off of pain medications and rehabilitated before the surgery, the majority would have obtained enough relief from their original problem to avoid the surgery all together.

Scar tissue is also a cause of failed back syndrome. Scar formation is a normal healing process following any surgery on the body. Most scars on our skin are not painful unless a nerve is injured and forms a neuroma (enlargement of the end of a cut nerve, which may be painful or may not). The same is true for spine surgery. It is rare to see an injured nerve as the cause of failed back surgery. Scarring around the spinal nerves following surgery is rarely the cause of the pain. The exception is when the scar tightly attaches a spinal nerve to an adjacent disc or facet joint. When this happens the nerve can be repeatedly stretched by abnormal motion in the degenerated unstable disc. One of the rationales for performing spinal fusion is to prevent this from happening by immobilizing the abnormal disc space.

Another thing that I have seen blamed on scar tissue as the reason for failed back surgery is that a partially cut ligamentum flavum (the yellow ligament between the lamina which is cut in every laminectomy) can bunch up and compress or stretch a spinal nerve. This is a common cause for failed micro-discectomy where portions of the ligament are cut but not completely removed. The entire cut portion of the ligament is removed during a standard discectomy so that retained ligament is not a problem following this procedure.

Failed disc surgery

There are several other reasons why failed back syndrome can occur following disc excision. I have surgically removed a fragment of disc the size of your thumb and was sure there were no more fragments to remove. On closer inspection, I have found another fragment of disc the same size as the first one! This happens more often than you would think. When a disc herniation is composed of several large fragments, there is reported to be a 25 percent risk of a recurrent disc herniation at the same site at a later date. This happens no matter how carefully the first surgery was performed. Fortunately, most disc herniations are not large and/or fragmented and are associated with less than a 5 percent risk of re-herniation following surgical removal.

Discs can herniate on the opposite side at the same level as the first disc excision and at other levels (remember the example of the young doctor who had disc herniations at three different levels at different times).

Normally patients have immediate relief of leg and arm pain following a disc excision. If the same pain persists immediately following surgery, then a retained disc fragment should be suspected. Retained fragments of disc can usually be detected with another MRI scan. If the extremity pain goes away for a period of time but then recurs in the same distribution and character as before, a recurrent disc herniation at the same site as before should be suspected. However, when the pain is in a different distribution than that experienced before the surgery, a disc herniation should be suspected at a different level than was operated upon.

Spinal stenosis and failed back syndrome

Following disc excision in the low back, the disc space can continue to narrow and cause spinal stenosis. The most common level for this to occur at in the low back is at the L5-S1 disc space. The disc excision provides relief of the stabbing pain and numbness down the leg to the bottom and side of the patient's foot. Removing the disc herniation relieves the symptoms from the compressed S1 nerve root. As the disc continues to degenerate and narrow, the L5 nerve root becomes entrapped in its passageway nearby. The patient then begins to experience a diffuse aching sensation down the same side of both legs while walking, but the pain is relieved by sitting, which is classical neurogenic claudication from spinal stenosis (see page 75). The pain may radiate to the top of the foot rather than the side and bottom of the foot prior to the disc surgery. I try to prevent this from happening by enlarging the passageways for the nerves (foramenotomy) when I perform a disc excision. It is hard to do this through a small incision, which is one reason I think a standard incision rather than a micro-incision is a better way to remove a disc herniation (see page 61).

Spinal instability causing failed back syndrome

Approximately 20 percent of people will experience chronic mechanical low-back pain following removal of a herniated disc. In fewer than 5 percent of people these symptoms will become so disabling as to warrant being labeled as failed back syndrome and require a spinal fusion for relief. It does not seem wise to perform a spinal fusion on everyone who undergoes a disc excision in order to prevent only 5 percent from having a second operation. When I explain this to my patients who are about to have a disc excision, they agree — no fusion.

Missed diagnosis or more than one source of pain as cause of failed back syndrome

Six weeks following an L5-S1 disc excision, one of my patients was still complaining of leg pain and still had a strongly positive straight-leg-raising test (see page 51). She also complained that she could not sleep because of the pain. I suspected a recurrent disc herniation and ordered a new MRI scan with contrast dye. Much to my amazement, she had a tumor at the L4-5 level, but the old disc herniation at L5-S1 was gone compared to her original MRI scan. There was no sign of a tumor on her original MRI scan, which had been performed without contrast dye. A neurosurgeon colleague of mine removed her benign tumor, resulting in excellent long-term relief. She definitely had two problems, an L5-S1 disc herniation and a tumor at the L4-L5 level of her spine. I do not know if both problems were causing her pain or whether the disc herniation was asymptomatic (see Chapter 5) and only the tumor was causing the pain. This case illustrates another reason for failed back syndrome, missed diagnosis or multiple diagnoses.

There are also several ways that failed back syndrome can occur following surgery for spinal stenosis. Remember from Chapter 6 on spinal stenosis that there are five places at each level of the lumbar spine where a nerve can be entrapped. A single or several nerves may be entrapped at several levels and sites at the same time. Sometimes it is very difficult to detect all of the places of nerve entrapment at the time of surgery. Failure to decompress all of the sites of entrapment can be a reason of failed back syndrome. This can be avoided by using a high-quality MRI scan to identify all of the places of entrapment prior to surgery (see discussion on closed MRI in Chapter 5, page 52). The first surgery may be adequately performed, with the patient experiencing relief of pain and resuming walking normally, only to have the symptoms of spinal stenosis recur. When this sequence of symptoms occurs, the spinals stenosis has either recurred at the same level or affected another level of the spine. This occurs in fewer than 5 percent of cases, and I do not know of any way to prevent it from happening.

Just as a herniated disc and spinal stenosis can recur, so can a facet joint cyst (illustrated on page 78). Recurrence of these conditions alone or together may be a cause for failed back syndrome. By now you undoubtedly have a better appreciation of how complex the spine is and how difficult the judgments are that must be made for surgical treatment of back pain the first time and certainly for failed back syndrome.

Adjacent segment disease as a cause of failed back syndrome

One of the most common reasons for failed back syndrome is adjacent segment failure, which is breakdown of the disc, ligament, and/or bone at a level proximal or distal to a spine fusion. I had recommended to a patient a decompression of multiple-level spinal stenosis and fusion with metal fixation to correct a complex deformity (slippage, tilting forward, and curvature) at four levels between L2 and the sacrum. The patient e-mailed me a copy of a paper entitled "Adjacent Segment Failure above Lumbosacral Fusions Instrumented to L1or L2" that was posted on the Internet. The author's conclusion that long instrumented fusions were unacceptable because of a 30 percent rate of failure frightened my patient. My response to the patient was as follows: "The problem is that this extensive surgery is performed for people with extensive problems such as yours. You have curvature (scoliosis), slippage at two levels (degenerative spondylolisthesis), constriction (spinal stenosis), and osteoporosis of the spine. For you to obtain relief of pain and regain function requires a decompression of the constricted areas of your spine and stabilization with a fusion from L2 to the sacrum. If you do not have surgery I think your condition will gradually become worse and surgery will be more difficult. However, there is a 25 percent risk that you will require additional surgery at some time in the future because of the nature of your condition."

Adjacent segment disease occurs because of two problems. Stress on the spine is shifted from a fused disc space to adjacent unfused levels. If the adjacent unfused discs or bony structures are predisposed to break down, they will not hold up to the increased stress. This is usually the case in patients who require fusions in the first place. It is difficult to predict who will develop adjacent segment disease following a spinal fusion and therefore how many levels to include in a spinal fusion. I have seen this problem require a second operation in fewer than 20 percent of my patients.

Failed back surgery can be caused by operating on the wrong level, incomplete surgery on the correct level, operating for the wrong diagnosis, and, when there are multiple sources of pain, failing to correct all of them at the time of surgery. It can also develop because of the nature of the disease. I have given you examples of each reason why back surgery fails.

Unmet expectations of surgery outcome as a reason for failed back syndrome

I get this joke from my patients all the time: "Doc, since the surgery I can't play the piano anymore." To which I reply, "I am sorry, why is that?" And the patient answers, "Oh I couldn't play it before the surgery either!"

Finally, back surgery can fail simply because the patient's expectations were not met. Both you and your doctor must have a clear understanding of what the expected outcomes of the surgery are. You have an obligation to tell the doctor what your expectations from the surgery are, and your doctor has an obligation to tell you whether she or he can meet those expectations. I frequently tell patients that there is a high probability that the surgery will relieve their pain and improve the quality of their life but a low probability that they will be able to perform certain activities such as skiing, running, playing tennis, or, in some cases, golfing. It is best for both parties to have a clear understanding of these issues before the surgery to avoid a feeling that the surgery has failed when unrealistic expectations are not met.

CHAPTER 11

How to Prevent Back Pain From Ruling Your Life

> ***How can I keep from having back pain again? How can I control the chronic pain that I have? How can I keep from getting bent over when I get older like my grandmother? How can I keep my children from suffering like I have from back pain?***

I was in my late 20s when I had my first attack of back pain. I realized that I was not taking good care of myself. I had been a college lacrosse player but stopped exercising regularly after graduation. I also made the big mistake of taking up smoking – during medical school, no less! With a combination of sitting in classes for long hours, lack of exercise, smoking, and a family history for bad backs, it was inevitable that I would suffer an attack of back pain.

Although I had already stopped smoking by the time of my first back-pain attack, I had not yet resumed exercising. I vowed to begin a lifetime of exercise so that I would never suffer like that again. My father, who lived a sedentary life and smoked, suffered repeated attacks of back pain, whereas my mother, who exercised daily and did not smoke, never had back pain. I began to emulate my mother, and started exercising on a regular basis. To this day I have a propensity for backaches, but I have never suffered from a disabling attack like my first attack of back pain. My wife and I walk four miles several days a week, and I am also otherwise physically active. My MRI scan shows that I have multiple degenerated discs in my spine.

The medical literature substantiates what I have personally experienced and what I have observed from my patients: staying physically fit and not smoking are the two best things you can do to decrease the frequency and severity of back-pain attacks. It is that simple; and you have complete control over your own destiny!

Everyday things to avoid in order to prevent back pain

There are a few other suggestions regarding your everyday activities that will help keep you from having an attack of pain. There are certain activities that can bring on attacks of neck and back pain that may not have occurred to you. You may not associate these activities with your pain because it frequently does not come on until a day or two after doing them. One of these is sitting on the floor. When I sit on the floor and play with my grandchildren, I invariably will develop back pain a day or two later. Other activities that will do this are lifting heavy travel bags into the overhead compartments of airplanes or, even worse, lifting bags off the carousels in baggage claim. Usually this requires that you quickly snag a heavy bag (if it was light you would have carried it on) and then twist as you lift. Lifting a heavy object while twisting and being off balance is a very bad move for your back.

It has been shown that, to prevent back pain, children should avoid carrying heavy book bags. Weight lifting is not good for children and adolescents, and hyperextension sports such as gymnastics are associated with back pain in adolescence.

Sleeping on your stomach can bring on neck pain, particularly if you are not accustomed to doing this. I have found that sleeping in this position is more difficult as I get older and develop more degenerative changes in my neck. Looking up for any extended period of time, such as by sitting too close to the stage in the theater, cleaning ceilings in your kitchen, or watching overhead fireworks, can bring on attacks of neck pain. Conversely, I almost always develop neck pain after reading an interesting book for a few hours at a time while lying in bed with my neck flexed. Many of these and similar activities are not associated with attacks of back pain because they do not hurt at the time you are doing them. The pain comes on a few days later.

Exercise: the best preventive medicine for back pain

You cannot prevent the fact that you are human and that our species is prone to disc degeneration and back pain. However, you *can* stack the odds in your favor by keeping in shape. My surgery resident had three disc herniations requiring three operations before the age of 26. Despite having such a bad back, he stays in shape and enjoys an excellent quality of life.

In Chapter 9 I went over three clinical studies that substantiate the benefits of exercise for the treatment and prevention of acute and chronic back pain, but why does it work? It seems to work in three different ways.

First, exercise contributes to the healthy nutrition of the cells in your discs. Remember how the nutrients diffuse into your discs, and waste is squeezed out (Chapter 1)?

Second, it is known that controlled exercise stimulates your body to rebuild injured parts faster than rest does. Years ago a sprained ankle was treated in a cast for six weeks, following which it took forever to rehabilitate the ankle. Today we treat sprained ankles in functional braces for protection so that you can "walk it off." It now takes half the time to return to full activity following an ankle sprain. The same thing is true for acute and chronic back pain. Controlled exercise makes the discs and ligaments in your spine heal faster.

Finally, exercise stimulates your endorphins, which in turn enhances healing. Exercise, exercise, exercise is the answer to prevention of acute and chronic back pain. The same reiteration applies to not smoking.

How does quitting smoking help prevent back pain?

Why is smoking so bad for your back? How does it increase the likelihood of suffering from acute and chronic back pain? Let's first explore the bad things that smoking does to your body in general, and then to your back in particular.

Some of the multiple toxic chemicals in cigarette smoke are potent immunosuppressive agents. Smoking the equivalent of one pack of cigarettes a day is like voluntarily taking cancer chemotherapy drugs. No one would do that voluntarily! They suppress your own body's normal defense mechanisms. This is why smokers are much more apt to develop post-operative wound infections than non-smokers. Second, some of these toxic chemicals inhibit normal wound healing. That is why plastic surgeons insist that their patients stop smoking before having plastic surgery. The inhibition of healing applies to all of the connective tissues in your body: bone, ligaments, skin, tendons, and yes, spinal discs!

As if suppression of your immune system and inhibition of healing were not enough, smoking also asphyxiates your tissues! The carbon monoxide in tobacco smoke attaches to your red blood cell hemoglobin (the red chemical in your blood that carries oxygen from your lungs to your body) more firmly than oxygen. Ten percent of pack-a-day smokers' hemoglobin bonds to carbon monoxide, which makes their red blood cells less able to carry oxygen from their lungs to their discs. When your spinal discs are robbed of oxygen, the cells die and leak painful chemicals into your disc. Both acute and chronic back pain is made worse by the toxic effects of tobacco smoke as the result of a combination of these factors.

There isn't *any* way that smoking is good for your back or for the rest of your body, for that matter! Smoking is responsible for an increased risk of almost every known form of cancer: lung, stomach, breast, prostate, bladder, bowel, and many others. Ladies, smoking causes premature wrinkles and osteoporosis. Gentlemen, smoking causes heart disease and premature impotency. If this litany of horrors doesn't convince you to quit smoking or never take it up, I don't know what will!

If you are a non-smoker, don't even think about starting if you want to be free of back pain. If you smoke, quit as soon as you read these words. In my experience with helping hundreds of smokers successfully stop, the best way to quit is cold turkey. It takes two weeks for the nicotine cravings to subside, and in six months you will hate the smell of tobacco smoke. It has been my observation that people who substitute nicotine patches, gum, and/or food have a higher relapse rate than the folks who just stop. Try to convince a lady who gains weight when she stops smoking not to resume the habit! That is why I also recommend going on a diet at the same time you quit smoking.

A late relative of mine was a heavy smoker and finally quit late in life when she developed terrible back and leg pain from severe spinal stenosis. I advised her that the pain would go away within 48 hours if she stopped smoking. She stopped, the pain went away as predicted, and she was relatively comfortable for the remaining days of her life. When the carbon monoxide from the cigarette smoke cleared out of her system, more oxygen was able to get to the nerves in her constricted spinal canal, and that was enough to relieve her pain. Unfortunately, she quit smoking too late in life and subsequently died from emphysema.

How do I keep from getting crooked like my grandmother?

How can you keep from having painful deformity (kyphosis and scoliosis, see Chapter 7) of the spine as you get older? Start young, and advise your children and grandchildren to do the same. Never smoke, and if you do, stop now. Smoking is one of the most potent causes of osteoporosis because it turns off the bone-building cells, the osteoblasts. Smoking also inhibits the absorption of calcium from your gastrointestinal system. Excessive intake of alcohol and caffeine will also do this and should also be avoided. The combination of bone-building cells that don't work and no calcium to work with weakens the vertebrae in your spine.

Osteoporosis and back pain

Weight-bearing exercises, like walking and light weight lifting, stimulate your bone-forming cells to make stronger bones. An adequate intake of calcium and Vitamin D (minimum of 1,000 mg calcium/day and 1,000 IU vitamin D) are also necessary for strong bones. A lifetime of regular exercise and adequate calcium and vitamin D are the two most important things you can do to ward off osteoporosis, painful vertebral fractures, and deformity of the spine.

For women who have premature menopause, that is, they lose their ovarian function at a younger-than-average age, it is important to have adequate estrogen replacement until the time of normal onset of menopause, in the early 50s. Estrogen replacement is not as important after menopause for the prevention of osteoporosis. Since estrogen replacement is also associated with a slight increase in risk of blood clots in the legs, lungs (pulmonary embolus) and brain (stroke), it is no longer recommended for prevention of osteoporosis after menopause. However, the decision for estrogen replacement should be made in consultation with your primary care physician or gynecologist.

Those at risk for osteoporosis (small postmenopausal women, smokers, former smokers, non-exercisers, women who entered menopause prematurely, people on steroids and/or with chronic diseases, coffee drinkers, and those who consume heavy amounts of alcohol) should have a BMD (bone-mineral density) test performed. This test determines how much calcium you have in your spine. The results can predict your risk of developing a painful deforming vertebral fracture. Depending on the results of the BMD test, you may need to be treated with medications that increase the strength of your bone and decrease the risk of painful vertebral fractures. There are a number of effective medications available for this purpose. Your PCP can help you select the one that is right for your circumstances.

How about a corset or brace to prevent my back pain?

There was a time when you would see every salesperson in home repair stores wearing a weight lifter's belt to prevent back injuries. A combination of soft science and clever marketing had convinced many employers to provide their workers with weightlifter's belts. Subsequent well-designed clinical studies demonstrated that these belts did nothing to prevent back injuries and the belts disappeared overnight. The employers should have read about the Los Angeles firefighters (see Chapter 9, page 120). The firefighters who remained physically fit were less apt to injure their back on the job. Employers would be much smarter to encourage their workers to work out regularly and stay in shape. Once again, the best way to prevent back pain is to keep fit.

How to keep whiplash of the neck from destroying your life

While we were walking one day, my wife pointed out an advertisement on the back of a Miami-Dade bus which read: "Automobile Accident Clinic, We help you with your pain, we work with your lawyer." I have observed over the years that one of the biggest impediments to relief from neck and back pain as the result of an auto accident is a combination of medical treatments and legal advice on how much the injury is worth. This is particularly true when the doctor and the lawyer work together, which is a potentially bad combination for you. You can be assured that their interest is to make sure your pain is disabling and your treatment is extensive, expensive, and lasts until your case is settled. Unfortunately you may have lost your job, your family (because they cannot stand your complaining any longer), become hooked on narcotics, and become so depressed in the process that life is not worth living. Not infrequently the unnecessary medical expenses, legal fees, and lawyer's contingency fees leave nothing from the settlement for you. Even worse is that your painful injury would more than likely have resolved itself if it had been left untreated! Instead, you are left with an unresolved chronic pain syndrome and you no longer have access to the doctor and lawyer who were manipulating your case.

The good news is that the most common, painful, demoralizing, and otherwise troubling spinal injury – whiplash to your neck from a rear-end collision – is rarely a serious injury today. Although it is one of the most aggravating and anxiety-producing injuries that you can sustain to your spine, it is usually self-limiting and requires minimal treatment for relief.

When you bend your neck forward you can only go far enough for your chin to strike the front of your neck. When you bend your neck backward, the only restraint are the ligaments in front of your spine. The term whiplash refers to an injury to the neck that occurs as the result of a rear-end collision. If you are a passenger in a car that is struck from behind, your neck will suddenly be whipped backward. In older cars that aren't equipped with proper headrests that restrain how far backward your neck is whipped, you can sustain terribly disabling sprains of the ligaments, muscles, and even discs in the front of your neck. The whiplash injury's awful reputation is a result of the severe hyperextension injuries passengers in such older cars have suffered in rear-end collisions.

For the past 20 years, with the advent of proper headrests that are positioned properly behind and close to your head, the severity of whiplash injuries has decreased dramatically. I have seen patients who were riding in cars that were struck so hard from the rear that the whole back of the passenger seat was broken, and yet they were not severely injured. The headrest kept their head in line with their body, thus preventing a sudden whiplash of their neck.

Why is it so common for people who suffer a whiplash injury of their neck to sue for pain and suffering? There are several reasons. The injury is usually brought on by someone who was not paying attention while driving, and the way it occurs makes the victim feel vulnerable and angry. They do not see it coming, and it frightens them. The symptoms of whiplash can be most aggravating, including headache, nausea, neck pain, difficulty sleeping, and anxiety. If they are treated with an immobilization collar, bed rest, massage, manipulation, and narcotic pain medication, the symptoms will linger forever. On the other hand, if they walk it off, use heat and/or ice, whichever works best, and anti-inflammatory medication, the chances are that the symptoms will subside completely within a matter of four to six weeks. It is difficult to follow this approach if your doctor and your lawyer are telling you that you are seriously injured and that you should be compensated for your pain and suffering.

Whiplash injury of the neck is essentially a sprain of the muscles, ligaments, and sometimes discs in the front of your neck. We have learned from treating sprained ankles that walking them off hastens healing. The same is true for a neck sprain. A soft collar may help for a day or two, but a hard plastic collar only makes things worse by inhibiting healing. The best way to get quick relief from the majority of whiplash injuries is to walk them off.

Is there ever a time when a whiplash injury is dangerous and you should not try to walk it off? There are two situations in which you should seek expert help from a qualified orthopaedist, neurosurgeon, neurologist, or physiatrist. Any older person with a history of neck pain may have spinal stenosis. When spinal stenosis narrows the spinal canal and constricts the spinal cord, a further sudden narrowing of the spinal canal from a whiplash injury can injure the spinal cord and cause a form of injury to the spinal cord called central cord syndrome, in which the arms may become weak but the legs are spared. Any feeling of weakness in the arms or legs following a whiplash injury should be diagnosed immediately. If you have a sensation of pins and needles or stabbing pain in the arms or legs with bending your neck forward following such an injury, it is a sign that the spinal cord has been injured and you should seek help. Do not keep testing for these symptoms if they occur once; just seek expert help right away. If you have immediate onset of severe neck pain and difficulty swallowing following a motor vehicle accident, or if you were knocked unconscious, then you should seek help. Sometimes it is not apparent immediately following an accident of any sort that you have sustained a serious neck injury; therefore, if any of these symptoms should come on later, ask for help.

Remember to question the real necessity of treatments such as narcotics, muscle relaxants, repeated manipulations, and hard plastic collars for a whiplash. Beware of the doctor or chiropractor who encourages you to see his lawyer associate. Most legitimate doctors whom I know refrain from referring their patients to a lawyer because they feel it is a conflict of interest to be involved in your legal case related to a motor vehicle accident. Good doctors are your advocate and want you to have the most effective, safest, and least expensive treatment. They do not want to be in conflict with your lawyer. They can best watch out for your interest if they are not associated with your lawyer. Most lawyers are ethical and also want the same thing for you, and they can function better if they do not have a relationship with the doctor. These issues are important for your health, particularly when it comes to whiplash injuries of the neck.

I have seen many patients through the years who are suffering from chronic back pain syndromes as the result of too much and too many types of treatment. They are cured by stopping all treatment and by not seeing doctors anymore! This has led me to believe that many people could avoid suffering from chronic back pain by avoiding certain treatments and too much treatment. For example, if you want to avoid chronic pain, never let your doctor place you on strong narcotics (see Chapter 8). Never go to bed for more than a day or two for back pain. Don't have repeated "maintenance" adjustments of your spine (Chapter 9). Don't have a spinal fusion for back pain caused by degenerative disc disease, especially if it was diagnosed by a discogram (Chapter 8). For that matter, don't have a discogram. Clinical studies show that people with discogenic back pain do better with exercise than with spinal fusion. Don't become dependent on any treatment. Always have a plan with your doctor to stop any treatment at an appropriate time. If you suffer from depression along with back pain, seek out treatment for the depression from your primary care physician, not a pain management specialist or spinal surgeon. Exercise, don't smoke or drink excessively, and watch your weight. These are some ways to prevent suffering from chronic back pain.

What about sex and back pain?

I saw a young man in my clinic two and a half months after I had performed a spinal fusion on his low back. He was accompanied by his wife. He informed me that he had been working since a month following the surgery and that he had some good news. His wife blushed as he informed me that she was pregnant with their first child. I congratulated them and inquired how far along she was in her pregnancy. She said as best they could tell around two months. He said that they were sure she conceived shortly after he had come home from the hospital following his spinal fusion! He said he wanted to make sure "it" still worked following the spinal fusion. We all had a good laugh, the story made my day, and they agreed that I could relate it to you as a segue into the subject of sex and back pain. I am not telling you that you should be able to have normal sex so soon after a spinal fusion, since their case is the exception, but I am saying that often the inability to have sex while suffering from a painful spinal condition may be secondary to fear, anxiety, or over-precautionary advice from your doctor, and not from the actual condition.

In the 1980s a colleague of mine wrote a book on back pain for the general public, which contained a whole chapter on sex. The chapter was replete with line drawings of couples having sex in various positions to illustrate how to avoid exacerbating a painful back condition. I am sure that this chapter helped sell a lot of books, but I am not sure it was completely necessary or particularly helpful to the readers. I am sorry to tell you that there will be no illustrations to accompany this discussion, but only helpful advice on how to enjoy a normal sexual experience despite suffering from back pain. There will also be some hints on how not to aggravate back pain while enjoying sex.

On the questionnaire that I have patients fill out regarding their back pain before they are seen in my clinic, there is a question concerning difficulty with sex. Most of the people who answer this question in the affirmative have multiple medical problems such as depression, obesity, hypertension, and/or diabetes in addition to their painful spinal condition. Most otherwise-healthy people, with the exception of people who have medical-legal issues (as discussed earlier in this chapter under "How to keep whiplash of the neck from destroying your life"), do not have difficulty with sex despite a painful back. It is my observation that "difficulty with sex" is a problem that is associated with general health and emotional issues more than with painful spinal conditions.

It is known that male smokers lose their libido at a relatively early age. Obesity, lack of exercise, diabetes, and hypertension are associated with a loss of interest in sex. When a person complains of "difficulty with sex" because of back pain, more often than not the problem is related to some other health issue such as depression, diabetes, smoking, obesity, and/or medications rather than the painful back condition per se. Successful rehabilitation of the individual usually corrects the libido problem. Restoration of a normal sex life is a good incentive to lose weight, exercise, stop smoking, and stop taking pain medications. All of these measures also relieve back pain.

What if you have a chronic back problem such as spinal stenosis and having sex aggravates your pain? How can you satisfy your partner and at the same time be satisfied from lovemaking in the face of a chronic painful spine condition? Here are some hints. Determine the movements that aggravate your pain. For example, with spinal stenosis, arching your back can aggravate neck and back pain. When this happens to a man, the best way to prevent it is to assume the bottom position during intercourse. In this way he can keep his neck and low back in a flexed posture. Lying on the side is also an option.

Women with spinal stenosis in the low back may find it more comfortable to assume the top position during intercourse. Also, spreading the legs can aggravate the symptoms of spinal stenosis. Women who suffer from spinal stenosis may find that lying on the side and having their partner approach from behind is the most comfortable and satisfying way of having intercourse. The woman does not need to arch her back or spread her legs during this approach.

Except in rare circumstances, sex is safe if you can find a comfortable position and your partner understands and accommodates your needs. Unless your doctor has specific reasons why you should not participate in sex, you can find a way if you have the will.

In my experience, wearing a brace, sleeping on a special bed, sitting in a special chair, or a using a disabled parking sticker will not prevent you from having chronic back pain. Only regular exercise, not smoking and drinking excessively, and watching your weight will prevent you from suffering from chronic back pain. The really great news is that these measures really work, they are totally under your control, and they are affordable!

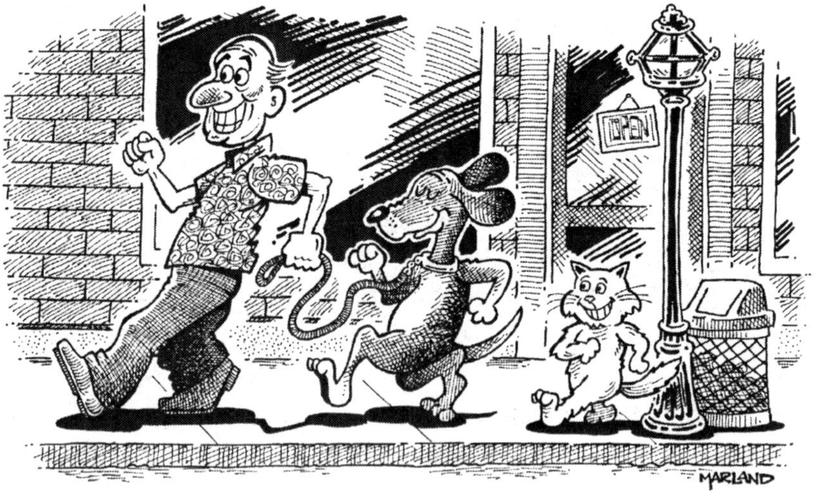

CHAPTER 12

Disc Transplants, Replacements, and Gene Therapy: They Sound Good, But Do They Work?

The exciting new approaches for treatment of back pain are focused on replacing or repairing a painful and worn-out disc. The three major approaches are: 1) to replace the worn-out disc with an artificial disc; 2) transplant a healthy disc to replace the worn-out disc; or, 3) repair the disc using gene therapy.

Fusion of a disc space in the neck and low back is associated with accelerated breakdown of adjacent discs. In order to avoid this problem, it is theoretically advantageous to restore normal motion in the abnormal disc by replacing or repairing it.

Artificial discs are used to treat chronic disabling back pain secondary to disc degeneration.

Artificial hip and knee replacements work; why not have an artificial disc replacement?

Artificial disc replacement is the most developed of the attempts to restore the normal motion and weight bearing of a worn-out disc. In 2006, the first lumbar disc replacement was approved by the U.S. FDA. Throughout the world, more than 10,000 patients have had this model of artificial disc placed in their low back. There are at least 10 other models of artificial discs being used throughout the world. At a recent seminar on innovations in spine surgery, I heard several discussions concerning the artificial disc. During the meeting I wrote down the following notes regarding disc replacement: "limited indications, technically difficult to perform, potential life- and limb-threatening complications, fixing failures is difficult, if a spinal fusion is required to repair a failed procedure it is difficult to perform, and the results of the fusion are not as good as would be expected." I then heard a lecture from a spinal surgeon, whom I respect, on his experience with treating more than 100 patients with an artificial disc.

The ideal candidate for a lumbar disc replacement, according to this experienced surgeon, is a 40-year-old female who needs one moderately degenerated disc replaced because of back pain that has lasted more than one year despite treatment. She has no leg pain, is moderately active, and has not had previous surgery. In addition, the patient should be in good health, of normal weight, and a non-smoker. As you can imagine, there are very few people who fit into this description! He went on to say that people who are not good candidates for a disc replacement have some combination of the following: multiple degenerated discs; inactive lifestyle; overweight; have a herniated disc squeezed into the spinal canal causing leg pain; had previous abdominal or pelvic surgery; are over 60 years or under 21 years of age; is a smoker; and, have spinal stenosis, spondylolisthesis, scoliosis, facet joint arthritis, osteoporosis, or vascular disease. The list goes on! I know a lot more people who have one or more of these contraindications than I know who are ideal candidates for disc replacement.

I am a very experienced surgeon, and when I think a spinal operation is technically difficult, it truly is. And I think artificial disc replacement is a technically difficult operation. Every experienced spinal surgeon I talk to thinks so also. If the artificial disc is not perfectly placed, there is a high probability that it will migrate out of position. If it settles into the adjacent vertebral bodies, it will prevent any motion between them. If it migrates backward into the spinal canal it can cause leg pain or nerve damage.

Conversely, if it migrates forward it can damage the adjacent blood vessels. Exact positioning of an artificial disc requires very clear live x-rays (fluoroscopy). The big problem is that it is almost impossible to obtain clear x-ray images in the operating room if the patient weighs too much. It is also difficult to safely expose the disc to replace it in a heavy individual because the wound is so deep, and excessive fat limits the exposure of the disc. To replace a disc in the low back requires that the major arteries carrying blood to your legs and the veins that carry the blood back to your heart must be moved aside (aorta, iliac arteries and veins, and vena cava). In the process of retracting these vessels aside to expose the disc they can be torn or otherwise injured. Excessive bleeding, loss of blood supply to a leg, or blood clots to the lungs can occur. The consequences may be so severe that you could lose a leg or your life! Smokers, people with high blood pressure, older, and overweight individuals are prone to have blood vessels that are more susceptible to injury and clotting. It is for these reasons that these individuals are not good candidates for disc replacement.

Lower lumbar disc replacement in men is more challenging than in women because of a nerve that is adjacent to the discs that controls normal ejaculation during sexual intercourse. In the process of exposing the discs in the lumbar spine this nerve can be injured, resulting in the ejaculation of semen backward into the urinary bladder (retrograde ejaculation). This presents two problems: difficulty conceiving children and a loss of the normal pleasurable sensation of ejaculation. Men who are anticipating disc replacement must accept the fact that retrograde ejaculation can occur no matter how carefully the surgeon retracts the nerve. If they cannot live with the possibility of this complication, they should not have the procedure.

Careful exposure of the disc is important to avoid injury to the adjacent vessels and nerves as well as to be able to accurately place the artificial disc. The exposure is much more difficult if the patient has had previous surgery such as an appendectomy, hysterectomy, or a disc replacement. This brings me to the next problem with disc replacement surgery. If the artificial disc should migrate out of normal position, become infected, wear out, or break, it should be removed and either replaced or the resulting space fused with bone. If it is difficult to place an artificial disc in the first place, it is really difficult to take one out. The exposure is more difficult and the surrounding structures are harder to retract aside. Once the artificial disc is removed, it is more difficult to replace one properly and more difficult to perform a fusion with bone graft should that be necessary.

Given all of these possible difficulties, why even have an artificial disc? Artificial discs are used to treat chronic disabling back pain secondary to disc degeneration. An artificial disc is the only surgical alternative to spinal fusion for this condition. The theoretical advantage of an artificial disc is that it preserves the motion of the disc space, thus preventing adjacent discs from prematurely breaking down. This has not been proven yet. In a U.S. FDA-approved study, a group of patients who received an artificial disc was compared in a prospective randomized study to a group of patients who underwent an interbody fusion using a metal cage (see Chapter 7). The serious complication rate for both procedures was less than 5 percent, but the patients with the artificial discs were happier with their surgery and had better pain relief than the patients who were fused with the metal cages. I think this study would have been more convincing if the artificial disc was compared to a group of patients who performed an intensive exercise program. Remember the study I quoted in Chapter 9, in which patients with chronic discogenic back pain had a satisfactory outcome from intensive back exercises? If intensive exercise works just as well as artificial disc or metal cage fusions, why take the chances of the surgical options? Remember my patient who was advised by another doctor that she was an ideal candidate for a disc replacement who exercised instead and was cured? (See her email to me on page 123)

For the rare young, otherwise healthy patient with chronic back pain from one or two degenerated lumbar discs, artificial disc replacement is a reasonable option if an intensive exercise program has not worked. But the patient must not smoke, they must be of normal weight, and must not have undergone a previous abdominal surgery.

Most of what I have said about artificial disc replacement in the low back also pertains to the neck. Since most cervical disc herniations are performed from in front and require complete removal of the disc, a spinal fusion is normally performed after removing the disc. Intuitively, it makes more sense to replace a cervical disc with an artificial disc than with a bone plug. The discs in the neck are more mobile than they are in the rest of the spine, and maintenance of this mobility may be more important than in the low back to protect adjacent levels. The U.S. FDA approved two artificial discs for the neck in 2007. There are several other artificial discs being used in clinical trials in the United States at this time. The possible complications from disc replacement in the neck are identical to those that can be encountered in an intervertebral fusion in the neck (see Chapter 9). The indications and contraindications to disc replacement in the neck are similar to those outlined above for the lumbar spine.

I have not personally treated any patients with an artificial disc, but I have recommended it as an alternative treatment to a few highly selected patients. After hearing a candid discussion of the pros and cons of artificial disc replacement, every patient with whom I have had this discussion has elected not to have the procedure. I think the indications for this procedure are limited in the low back to a highly selected patient, the so-called ideal candidate, whereas there is more of an indication for the procedure in the neck. Artificial disc replacement is still an "investigational procedure" in the United States. Whether this procedure will equal the efficacy of hip and knee replacement remains to be determined through refinement of the indications, technique, and long-term follow-up of the results.

They can transplant kidneys and hearts; why not discs?

It is true that heart transplants work and save people's lives, so why can't they transplant discs and save people's backs? A heart transplant recipient must take immunosuppressant drugs for the remainder of their lives to prevent their body from rejecting the transplanted heart. There are a number of unwanted side effects from taking these drugs. But the risk of these side effects is better than the alternative, which is likely death. Would it be worth the risk of taking immunosuppressant drugs in order to receive a disc transplant? Probably not, but what if you didn't have to take pills to keep you from rejecting a transplanted disc? From the extensive experience of the University of Miami Tissue Bank with transplanting major joints (to save arms and legs from amputation in cases of bone cancer) we know that immunosuppressant drugs are not necessary to prevent rejection. It seems that the controlled freezing process (the same one used to preserve live sperm and eggs) used to preserve the bone–cartilage grafts alters them in such a way that the body does not reject them the way it does with organs such as hearts and kidneys. Disc grafts are composed of a small portion of the adjacent vertebrae and the entire disc itself. This bone–disc–bone graft is controlled-frozen immediately after being retrieved from a cadaver donor. The disc grafts are similar to bone cartilage grafts in that the controlled freezing decreases the chance that they will be rejected by the body they are placed in.

The disc grafts are scanned by MRI to determine that they are normal and do not have degenerative changes. When they are transplanted, the vertebral bone from the recipient heals to the bone on the grafted disc, thus re-establishing pathways of nutrition to the graft. During this healing process, the grafted disc is in jeopardy of starving from poor nutrition. This may result in rapid degeneration of the otherwise healthy grafted disc. For this reason, transplantation of large discs (lumbar spine) may be less likely to succeed than smaller discs (cervical spine). The smaller the disc, the more easily nutrients can penetrate and keep the cells alive while new pathways are being established. Small animal studies have demonstrated that it is possible to transplant small discs that continue to function normally. But will this work in humans with relatively larger discs? A group of patients in Hong Kong who have received cervical spine disc transplants were regularly monitored for up to four years. They have had relief of pain, maintenance of disc space height, and normal neck motion. There have been no other reports of successful disc transplants in the low back.

Even if disc transplantation techniques eventually become better than artificial disc replacement, the surgery for the two procedures is equally demanding and risky. Either approach has specific risks, such as wear and breakage of an artificial disc or premature breakdown and rejection of a transplanted disc. Investigation of disc transplantation is still in its infancy, so only time will tell if it is a reasonable approach to the treatment of painful degenerative disc disease.

Since disc degeneration is genetic, is there hope in gene therapy?

Good question. Genetically engineered bone-stimulating proteins (see BMP, page 96) are already available to stimulate fracture healing and spinal fusion. These are situations that require a stimulus of a specific cell function (bone production) for a short period of time (until the fracture heals or the bone fusion occurs).

In the case of the repair of a degenerative disc, the missing cell function must be replaced for the patient's entire lifetime. This means that the missing or defective genes that ultimately are responsible for disc degeneration must be replaced in the disc cells. First the genes must be identified, then they must be inserted into the disc cells, and the cells must live long enough to repair and maintain a normal functioning disc. So how can all of this be accomplished?

First of all, disc cells are around for a long time – maybe as long as we live. That is, you may be given your full complement of disc cells from the very beginning, and that is all you get. Therefore, genetically altered disc cells would be around long enough to favorably influence the disc.

Second, disc cells are trapped in a matrix where there is no blood circulation to whisk away injected genes.

Third, a number of missing or defective genes responsible for production and maintenance of normal disc tissue have been identified and can be replicated. Finally, there are ways of piggybacking these genes onto harmless viruses that can carry them inside of disc cells where they can be put to work.

Research bench studies and animal studies have shown that you can genetically influence defective disc cells to produce a normal connective-tissue matrix. Test-tube studies are now in progress to determine the safest and most effective ways of transferring genes into human disc cells. I suspect that practical gene therapy to repair degenerated discs is just around the corner. In the meantime, nothing beats taking care of your own discs by exercising and avoiding those things (such as smoking and lack of exercise) that I have mentioned before!

Despite these remarkable new ideas for treating back pain, the best, safest, and most cost-effective cure is under your control. You and you alone can determine how you will take care of that remarkable engine, your body, and in particular your back, so that it will last a lifetime. You and you alone can prevent your suffering from back pain. The biggest breakthrough in treatment and prevention of back pain resides in your understanding of the problem and how you can solve it through good health habits.

I hope this book has helped you understand your problem and to find the best and safest way to "conquer back and neck pain".

–Dr. Mark Brown, Miami, Florida

Glossary

acupuncture: An elaborate oriental method that uses needles to stimulate specific anatomical sites under the skin to relieve pain

adjustments: A form of treatment in which the spine is passively manipulated; chiropractic method

ankylosing spondylitis: A form of arthritis of the spine that causes it to become stiff, brittle, and bent forward; sometimes referred to as "bamboo spine" because of its appearance on x-ray

annulus fibrosus: The tough, outer rim of the spinal disc that contains the spongy center (nucleus pulposus)

anterior interbody spinal fusion: Spinal fusion that is performed from the front of the spine, with a bone graft replacing the entire spinal disc

anti-coagulants: Medications that interfere with normal blood clotting; aspirin, most anti-inflammatory medications, Coumadin, vitamin E, and Plavix are the most common

aortic aneurysm: A blowout of the major blood vessel that leads from your heart to your body; depending on where it occurs, it can cause severe spinal pain; it can be a life-threatening condition

asceptic necrosis of the hip: Death of the ball portion of the hip joint; can occur from taking steroids by mouth as well as a number of other causes

banked bone: Bone that is taken from cadaver donors and stored in a tissue bank

BMD: *Bone mineral density:* a measurement used to detect osteoporosis

BMP: *Bone morphogenic protein:* a naturally occurring protein in your body that stimulates new bone formation; genetically engineered BMP is used to stimulate spinal fusion

bulging disc: Narrowed spinal disc that bulges circumferentially like a flat tire on a car

carpal tunnel syndrome: Pain and numbness in the hand caused by compression of the median nerve in the carpal tunnel of the wrist

CAT scan: Computer-assisted tomography: a diagnostic X-ray that provides a three-dimensional picture of the body part scanned

cauda equina: Cauda equina (literally means horse's tail in Latin) is the term applied to the multiple nerves that extend from the lower part of the spinal cord in the low back to your legs, your bowel, and your urinary bladder

cauda equina syndrome: Symptoms of severe back and leg pain associated with change in bowel and bladder function, numbness in the pelvic area, and loss of muscle strength in the leg(s) as the result of pressure on the cauda equina in the low back

central pain: A term coined by the author to describe a state of lowered threshold to pain secondary to altered pain modulation systems in the brain

cervical spine: That part of the spine that comprises the neck

chiropractic: Treatment method based upon a concept of joint misalignment (subluxation), particularly of the spine; practiced by chiropractors

chymopapain: An enzyme extracted from papaya fruit; it was widely used throughout the world to dissolve herniated discs

claudication: An aching, burning, and/or cramping sensation in the extremities brought on by activity; see neurogenic claudication and vascular claudication

claustrophobia: Fear of enclosed spaces

coccyx: The lower tip of the spine, "tail bone"

cosquillitas: Spanish meaning "little tickles"; a treatment method invented by the author to relieve musculoskeletal pain; works like acupuncture

COX-2 inhibitors: Anti-inflammatory medications that were designed to give pain relief with less risk of the bleeding and stomach irritation that are seen with other anti-inflammatory medication

disc degeneration: A condition in which the normal cushioning function of the spinal disc is lost through a process that is genetically determined

disc excision: Removal of that part of a herniated disc that is causing pain

discogenic pain: Pain arising from an abnormal spinal disc

discography/discogram: Diagnostic test in which x-ray contrast dye is injected into a spinal disc to determine the source of spine pain and the degree of disc degeneration

dura: Membrane that covers the brain, spinal cord, and origin of the spinal nerves; it contains the spinal fluid

electromyogram: see EMG/NCV

EMG/NCV: *Electromyogram and nerve conduction velocity:* a diagnostic test performed by placing needles in muscles and stimulating the nerves to the muscles; used to diagnose neuropathy and other neurological disorders

endorphins: Naturally occurring painkillers in the body

epidural hematoma: Hemorrhage into the space surrounding the brain or spinal cord; can be a complication of surgery, secondary to anti-coagulants, or from trauma; can result in nerve damage or paralysis

epidural steroid injection: Treatment method of injecting a small amount of local anesthetic and steroid medication directly into the area of the spine where a nerve is being irritated by a herniated disc

evidence-based medicine: Process through which the medical community determines the effectiveness and safety of a treatment based upon clinical research data

extruded discs: A disc herniation that has ruptured completely through the outer rim of the disc

facet joint cyst: Cyst on the facet joint that results from degenerative arthritis; these cysts are benign but can recur after being removed; they may cause symptoms of spinal stenosis

facet joints: Finger-sized joints that are located behind and to either side of each spinal disc and form the roof and walls of the spinal canal

facet rhizotomy: Treatment for back pain in which the sensory nerves to the facet joints are cut, frozen, poisoned, or destroyed with an electrical current

failed back syndrome: Recurring painful disorder after spinal surgery

femoral-stretch-test: A physical examination maneuver in which the patient is lying face down on a flat surface and the examiner bends the knee until pain is experienced in front of the thigh; most commonly seen with disc herniations in the low back

flat back: Loss of the normal concavity of the low back

fluoroscopy: X-ray technique in which real-time movement of the bony anatomy can be observed

foot drop: Weakness of the muscles that lift the foot off of the floor; can cause slapping of the foot on the floor while walking

foramenotomy: Surgical opening of the channels containing the spinal nerves

herniated disc (HNP): Associated with a tear in the rim of the disc (annulus fibrosus) with the center of the disc (nucleus pulposus) herniating through the tear.

IDET: *Intradiscal electro-thermal therapy:* a treatment for back pain in which the nerves near the spinal discs are cooked with a heating probe

idiopathic low back pain: Term for common attack of back pain in which the exact cause of the pain cannot be determined

kyphosis: Rounding of the spine as seen from the side; normally the chest has some kyphosis, but when it becomes abnormal the person looks as if they are hunched forward

L5-S1 disc: Spine disc between the 5th lumbar vertebra and the sacrum; usually the lowest disc in the low back, although some people have an L6-S1 disc and in some people the lowest disc is the L4-S1 disc

laminectomy: Removal of part of the roof of the spinal canal in order to view and remove a disc herniation

lordosis: The normal concavity of the low back when seen from the side

lumbar spine: That part of the spine that comprises the low back with the belly in front and surrounded behind and to the sides by muscles

Marfan's Syndrome: Inherited disorder characterized by tall stature and long thin figures and can cause severe spinal pain from rupture of the aorta (largest artery in the body)

meta-analysis: A medical research technique that involves a systematic review of a large number of peer-reviewed publications about a treatment

micro-surgery: Surgery that is performed through a small incision using a microscope at between 5 and 10X magnification

minimally invasive spine surgery: Description of a variety of surgical techniques of the spine that are performed through a small incision and/or arthroscopic type of devices

MRI: Magnetic Resonance Imaging: a diagnostic test that produces a picture of the body anatomy without X-ray exposure

myelogram: A diagnostic test in which X-ray contrast dye is injected into the spinal fluid in the spinal canal

myelopathy: A disease of the spinal cord that causes loss of balance, stumbling, aches and pains in the arms and legs, and propensity to fall

neurofibroma: Benign, slow-growing tumors of the nerves; can cause back pain with sleep disturbance

neurogenic claudication: Aching pain in the legs or arms aggravated by activity and relieved by rest; the result of constriction of the spinal nerves by spinal stenosis

neurogenic pain: Pain arising from stimulation of a nerve

neurologist: Medical specialist in diseases of the brain and spinal cord

neuropathy: Disease of the nerves in the extremities characterized by annoying sensations of numbness and tingling; usually associated with diabetes; affects the lower legs and feet

neurosurgeon: Surgical specialist in diseases of the brain and spinal cord

nucleus pulposus: The gelatinous spongy center of the spinal discs that distributes the weight of the spine; contained by the annulus fibrosis

orthopaedic surgeon: Medical and surgical specialist in bone, joint, and spine disorders

osteoid osteoma: Pea-sized benign bone lesion that can cause pin-point spine pain relieved dramatically by aspirin

osteophytes: Commonly called "bone spurs," bone projections that form on the edge of the vertebrae adjacent to a loose degenerated disc

osteoporosis/osteopenia: Literally means porous bones; a condition that results from not enough calcium in the bones

pain drawing: Front-and-back blank silhouette of the body on which patients draw symbols depicting the location and type of pain they are experiencing

pain management specialist: Medical doctors who treat acute and chronic pain disorders

Parkinson's disease/syndrome: Movement disorder that is associated with a tremor, rigid muscles and a shuffling gait

pars interarticularis: That part of the spine that attaches the facet joint to the pedicle; a defect in this structure is associated with slippage of the spine (spondylolisthesis)

pediatric orthopaedist: Orthopaedic surgeon who treats bone and joint diseases in children up to the age of 18; they usually treat scoliosis (curvature of the spine)

pediatrician: Doctor who treats children from birth to age of 18

pedicle: Bones that come off of the back of the spine vertebra on each side that act as the wall of the spinal canal and the attachment of the facet joints, lamina, spinous and transverse processes of the spine; this is the structure in which pedicle screws are placed

pedicle screws: Bone screws that are designed to be placed in the pedicles (walls) of the spine; they are attached to rods or plates to aid in spinal fusion

peripheral neuropathy: see neuropathy

physiatrist: Physical medicine and rehabilitation specialist who diagnoses and treats neruro-musculoskeletal disorders with special emphasis on rehabilitation

physical therapist: Health care provider who deals with assessment of neuro-musculoskeletal disabilities and the restoration of function using physical methods such as exercise

placebo: An inactive medicine or treatment used in controlled clinical research trials to compare to the treatment being tested

posterior interbody spinal fusion: Spinal fusion performed from behind, with bone graft replacing the entire disc

posterior lateral spinal fusion: Spinal fusion that is performed from behind and alongside the spinal canal

prolapsed disc: A herniated disc that has not ruptured completely though the outer rim of the disc

retrograde ejaculation: An abnormality of male sexual climax where the semen is projected backward into the urinary bladder rather than forward out of the penis; can be a complication from surgical exposure of the discs in the low back for an artificial disc replacement or fusion

rheumatoid arthritis: A form of arthritis that causes deformity of the hands and can cause serious instability of the spine in the neck

rheumatologist: Medical specialist in diagnosis and treatment of arthritis and other painful diseases of the bones, joints, and spine

rhizotomy: see facet rhizotomy

rotator cuff: Major muscle attachment for the muscles in the shoulder that commonly tears and causes pain

sacral spine: That part of the spine that attaches the spinal column to the pelvis

schwannoma: Benign, slow-growing tumors of the nerves; can cause back pain with sleep disturbance

sciatic nerve: The major nerve extending from the low back down the back of the leg and transmitting motor impulse to the muscles of the leg and sensation from the leg and foot to the brain

scoliosis: Abnormal curvature of the spine when viewed directly from the front or back, which is to be distinguished from the normal curves of the spine as seen from the side

sequestered discs: A disc herniation that has squirted completely into the spinal canal from the disc space

shingles (herpes zoster): Painful infection of a spinal nerve that is associated with a rash; the pain and rash run along the course of the nerve(s) involved and are the result of the chicken pox virus

shoulder-hand syndrome: Pain in the upper extremity that can be caused by several conditions, such as a disc herniation in the neck, shoulder arthritis, and/or carpal tunnel syndrome in the wrist

spinal discs: Cushions between the vertebrae of the spine that are composed of a gelatinous center (nucleus pulposus) and a fibrous rim (annulus fibrosus)

spinal fluid: Clear fluid that bathes the brain, spinal cord, and origin of the spinal nerves; it is contained by the dura

spinal headache: Headache that results from a spinal fluid leak; becomes intense when standing and is relieved by lying down; can be experienced after an epidural injection or spine surgery

spinal stenosis: Constriction of the spinal canal or foramen (passages for the spinal nerves)

spine fusion: Surgical union of spine segments; performed with or without metal screws and rods, and with bone graft from the pelvis or tissue bank

spondylolisthesis: Literally means slippage of the spine; one vertebra slips forward on the vertebra below; there are two types: 1) associated with an inherited defect in the bones behind the vertebrae (isthmic spondylolisthesis), and 2) associated with disc degeneration (degenerative spondylolisthesis)

straight-leg-raising test: A diagnostic physical exam maneuver in which the patient is lying face up on a flat surface and the leg is elevated by the examiner until pain is experienced; the degree of elevation of the leg is noted as well the extent of the pain from the back and down the leg; most commonly seen with herniated discs in the low back

stress X-rays: Bending X-rays of the spine which include a side-view while standing straight, while bent forward (flexion), and then while bending backward (extension) to detect abnormal motion (laxity or stiffness) of the spine

TENS: Transcutaneous electrical nerve stimulation: a treatment that uses specific electrical impulses applied to the skin to relieve pain

thoracic spine: That part of the spine with the ribs attached that comprises the chest

U.S. FDA: United States Food and Drug Administration: regulatory agency of the U.S. government that assures safety of drugs and devices

vascular claudication: Burning and/or cramping sensation in the legs or arms that is aggravated by activity and relieved by rest; it is caused by poor blood supply to the extremity

vertebra: The bone blocks that, along with the discs, make up the spinal column

vertebral fracture: A crack or break in a spinal bone block (vertebra)

whiplash injury: Refers to an injury to the neck that typically results from being a passenger in a vehicle that is hit from behind; the neck is suddenly whipped backward and forward

Index

CPSIA information can be obtained at www.ICGtesting.com
Printed in the USA
BVOW030422140812

297789BV00006B/13/P

9 781934 716472